AF598839

THE Artist's Mind

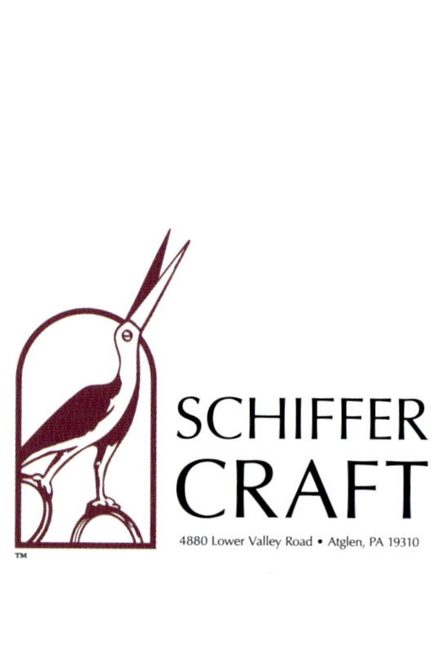
SCHIFFER
CRAFT
4880 Lower Valley Road • Atglen, PA 19310

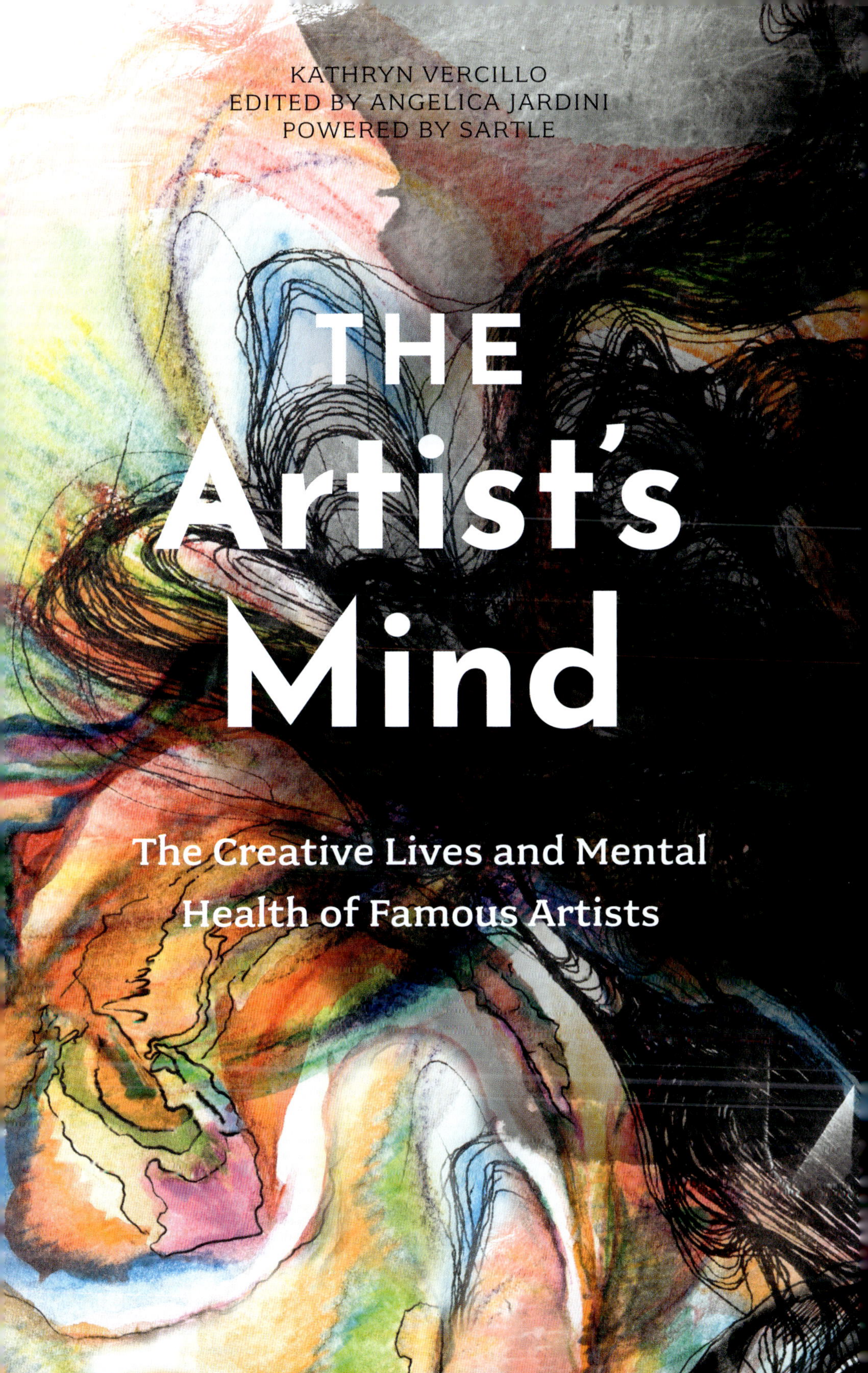
KATHRYN VERCILLO
EDITED BY ANGELICA JARDINI
POWERED BY SARTLE
THE
Artist's
Mind
The Creative Lives and Mental
Health of Famous Artists

OTHER SCHIFFER BOOKS BY THE AUTHOR:

Bad Blood: Rivalry and Art History, Clayton Schuster, Foreword by Noah Charney, Powered by Sartle, ISBN 978-0-7643-5730-5

Rogue Art History: The Trivia Game, Powered by Sartle, ISBN 978-0-7643-6178-4

Rogue Art History, National Portrait Gallery Edition: The Trivia Game, Powered by Sartle, ISBN 978-0-7643-6179-1

Other Schiffer Books on Related Subjects:

How Art Heals: Exploring Your Deep Feelings Using Collage, Andra F. Stanton, Foreword by Tien Chiu, ISBN 978-0-7643-6146-3

Intersection: Art & Life, Kevin Wallace, ISBN 978-0-7643-5519-6

Disrupted Realism: Paintings for a Distracted World, John Seed, Foreword by Katherine Stanek, ISBN 978-0-7643-5801-2

Library of Congress Control Number: 2021942421

Designed by Danielle D. Farmer
Cover design by Molly Shields
Illustrations by Tania Houtzager
Type set in Fairplex Wide OT/Josefin Sans

ISBN: 978-0-7643-6384-9
Printed in China

Published by Schiffer Publishing, Ltd.
4880 Lower Valley Road
Atglen, PA 19310
Phone: (610) 593-1777; Fax: (610) 593-2002
Email: Info@schifferbooks.com
Web: www.schifferbooks.com

This book is dedicated to you—the artist I may or may not know—who is living with challenging conditions of the mind and creates anyway. What you give to the world is important.

CONTENTS

— III —

— IV —

INTRODUCTION

"There's a fine line between madness and genius."

You've probably heard this idea before. But are artists really more likely than the rest of the population to struggle with mental illness? Do people with depression, anxiety, PTSD, OCD, or schizophrenia relate to the world in a way that allows them to see things uniquely and to express their vision of the world more artistically? What exactly is the relationship between mental health and artistic creativity? For decades, if not centuries, people have noticed some type of relationship between mental health and creative impulse, sometimes going so far as to exaggerate the connection.

There are countless myths, anecdotes, studies, surveys, and theories that try to capture this complicated topic. The truth is, we have only just begun to understand how the filaments of mental illness and the tendrils of creativity intertwine, cross paths, become parallel, and diverge.

Further troubling the subject, both mental illness and artistic inclination exist on their own spectrums. It's easy to classify people as being either in the category of "mentally ill" or "normal," but that's not the reality. Many people face some kind of mental health challenge at some point in their lives. Sure, at one end of the spectrum are the folks who have never had an experience with mental illness. At the other end are people born with serious disorders who may have psychotic breakdowns or difficulty functioning normally in the world. Most people, though, live somewhere in the middle. Take, for example, a new mother with postpartum depression, a teenager who struggles with an eating disorder, the successful businessperson with high-functioning anxiety, or an individual who goes through a traumatic experience and needs a few years of therapy and medication to work through that challenge. Each has unique experiences, symptoms, reactions, and perspectives on their issue, not to mention varied treatment solutions.

Then we have the *artistic* spectrum. At one end, you'll find people who have no interest in creative expression, and at the other are those who seem born to be artists. These people might start drawing, painting, writing, or singing before they can crawl—they are simply compelled to create art. Again, though, most people exist somewhere in the middle. Think of a working parent who loves to craft with their children, a person who makes art in their spare time while pursuing a non-art-related career, or someone who loved to draw as a child but hasn't done so in years. As with mental health, even people who seem to have similar stories will retain their own experiences, beliefs, creative processes, and relationship with their artistic practice.

So, **each of us lies somewhere on the mental health spectrum and somewhere on the artistic spectrum**. They overlap at different points and pull away at others; at times they may support each other but can also cause friction. As we look at the lives of artists throughout history who have navigated these convolutions, some questions we will explore and keep in mind are the following:

How might making art help with mental health symptoms?

How might making art trigger or exacerbate mental health symptoms? Are the pressures of making a living as an artist a factor?

And how do mental health challenges affect a person's ability to make art? Do their symptoms inspire them to create in new and innovative ways? Or do they struggle to make art while facing these challenges?

There are many answers to these questions, and certainly more than we will be able to cover in this book. When looking at a person's journey from the outside, no matter how objective and detailed the study, it is difficult—if not impossible—to grasp the full picture of their unique experience, especially for historical figures.

Yet, in musing upon the answers to these questions, we might come to better understand not only the wonderful art created by the people in this book, but also what is at the core of the human experience. Whether you're an artist or a person with a mental illness, an art historian or a psychology student, or just someone interested in the subjects of creativity and mental health, we hope that reading these stories will inspire you to think more broadly about the ways that art and mental health are connected.

In *The Artist's Mind*, we will share the life stories of twenty artists known to or believed to have lived with symptoms associated with mental health conditions. We look at artists on the depression spectrum, we discuss trauma (both individual and collective), and we explore schizophrenia and the concept of the "outsider artist," investigating the dynamics between artists with mental health issues and broader society.

In discussing different mental health issues, we will encounter a range of artists—people of different genders, cultures, and socioeconomic backgrounds from a variety of historical eras. That said, our studies were limited by the information available on historical figures. Although mental health challenges have become increasingly better understood over time, there remains a stigma. And while art history may be improving with inclusivity, there are still many stories missing from the canon. We recognize and acknowledge that what is offered here is just a starting point, and we hope that this book inspires others to seek further information about these fascinating subjects. Though it is far from exhaustive, we think that this collection of stories from artists' lives creates an intriguing picture of the nuanced ways in which mental health and creativity are linked.

As we look at the artists across history who have experienced mental health challenges, we must consider not only the specific obstacles each has had to overcome, but also when their illness might have even helped rather than hindered them. Each artist's experience with mental health and creativity is complex, nuanced, and highly individual. Ultimately, it is important to listen to what the individual themselves has to say, whether with their words or through their art.

A NOTE ON DIAGNOSIS

Diagnosing mental health conditions is complicated. Even in the twenty-first century, it's common for someone with symptoms to receive more than one diagnosis. Diagnosis is used to help doctors, therapists, and the individuals themselves better understand their symptoms, experiences, and treatment options. However, the science is messy. There's no blood test or brain scan that definitively says, "This is what you have." And, of course, diagnosis has changed significantly over time. It's informed not only by the medical understanding of the day but also by culture, philosophy, politics, religion, and other societal forces.

If Michelangelo or Vincent van Gogh were alive today, their experience would be different and their diagnoses would be different too. With many artists from the past, especially Van Gogh, twentieth- and twenty-first-century professionals have attempted a posthumous diagnosis. Obviously, if getting an accurate diagnosis is challenging when the client is right in front of you, it's nearly impossible when looking back at someone you've never met. So, we have to take historical diagnoses with a grain of salt, recognizing that although they can't accurately portray the artist's experience, they still provide us with useful information for discussing the relationship between mental health and the artistic process.

The artists explored in this book come from different eras. We note what that person's diagnosis was at the time, as well as what it might be considered today. **It's important to note two types of diagnoses from the past: those for conditions that still exist, and those that have fallen out of favor or have been completely dismissed.**

In the first category are conditions with a fairly comparable modern diagnosis. For example, we'll see that what we know today as schizophrenia was first called dementia praecox—two names for more or less the same constellation of symptoms. Another example is manic depression, an older name for what we now call bipolar depression. Also in this first category are historical conditions that are similar to a modern diagnosis but were seen through a very different lens. Melancholia is one example: it's a diagnosis comparable to dysthymia or major depression. However, the way that doctors and patients viewed melancholia differs greatly from our current understanding of the disorder. Let's use the artist Albrecht Dürer as a case study to explore these differences.

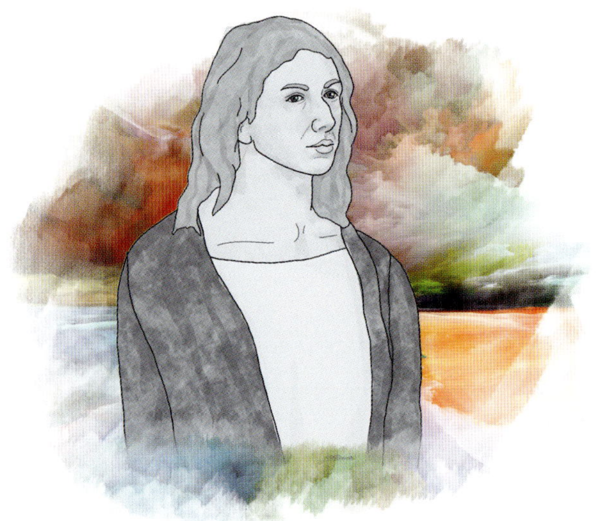

Albrecht Dürer

(May 21, 1471–April 6, 1528)

Albrecht Dürer created a powerful engraving, *Melancholia*, that some art historians have suggested is a self-portrait of his own depression. The title itself is a clue to the topic. Dark features, slouched posture, and the inclusion of symbols that represent depression help drive the point home. Melancholia was one of the "four humors," a system of understanding medicine that originated in ancient Greece. It was associated with black bile and depression, but also with creativity and art in Dürer's time. Researcher Jane Kromm explains:

> The melancholic character, originally one of the four humors and aligned over the years with the planet Saturn, altered in meaning during the late Middle Ages and Renaissance. In post-medieval poetry, melancholy became associated less with medical usage and increasingly with an emphasis on a subjective and transitory mood. . . . By the beginning of the Renaissance, this transitory nature was allied with a brooding withdrawal from reality. The heightened self-awareness that such a condition implied was tinged with the romantic connotation afforded a tragic hero. Moreover, melancholia came to be seen as an attractive condition.[1]

This perceived connection between the mind and body, and the subsequent romanticizing of melancholy, informed artists' perception of themselves and their work. We will see artists such as Frida Kahlo and Alice Neel, who specifically draw attention to the relationship between the physical body and mental health. Moreover, we'll see that many artists of the past, such as Francisco Goya and Edvard Munch, likely ascribed to the belief that their mental health symptoms and creativity derived from the same place.

Next is the second category of diagnoses: conditions that had a name and diagnostic criteria in the past but have no comparable diagnosis today. For example, neurasthenia, a condition regularly diagnosed in the nineteenth century, played an important historical role for women in general, and women artists in particular, before it fell out of favor. Neurasthenia was understood as a condition not entirely dissimilar to depression, with symptoms that included trouble sleeping and eating, physical aches and pains, and listlessness. However, it was specifically diagnosed in relation to the belief that "the harsh conditions of modern industrial society had generated new nervous disorders."[2] While both men and women might receive a diagnosis of neurasthenia, the suggested cure was deeply gendered; men were encouraged to get out of the city by adventuring outdoors or otherwise retreat into nature. Women, on the other hand, were instructed to go on complete bed rest and were often not allowed to read, write, or have visitors for weeks, or even months, on end.[3] Neurasthenia was primarily diagnosed from approximately 1870 to 1920, a time during which women's lives changed dramatically. They were out in public more, attending school, and now going to work. To that end, neurasthenia was most prevalently diagnosed in middle- and upper-class American women.[4] Thinking back to American history from this time, from the second wave of the Industrial Revolution to the First World War, it is not surprising that there were strong reactions to all the change and turbulence, all of which no doubt informed this diagnosis.[5]

Neurasthenia was a common diagnosis for decades, but society and medicine changed, and it's been about a century since it's been used. That said, depression is now a leading diagnosis in America, and many suggest that this condition, too, is a result of industrialization, technological advancements, and the alienation of modern life. So, even with these obsolete historical diagnoses, comparisons can be drawn to better understand what artists of the past may have experienced. For the purposes of this book, we will find it **useful to explore how diagnoses have shifted and evolved over time, always bearing in mind that an artist's mental health journey is undeniably influenced, at least in part, by time and place.**

AUTHOR'S NOTE

I have a master's degree in psychological studies from a program that integrated Eastern and Western psychology. I have used this education and experience to inform the discussions of mental health symptoms throughout this book. However, I am not a clinician and have not attempted to diagnose the artists discussed in this book. Instead, I've drawn both from the diagnoses recorded during the artist's lifetime and from posthumous diagnoses by recognized professionals who have been widely published. Finally, remember that a diagnosis is a helpful label or tool, but it doesn't define the individual.

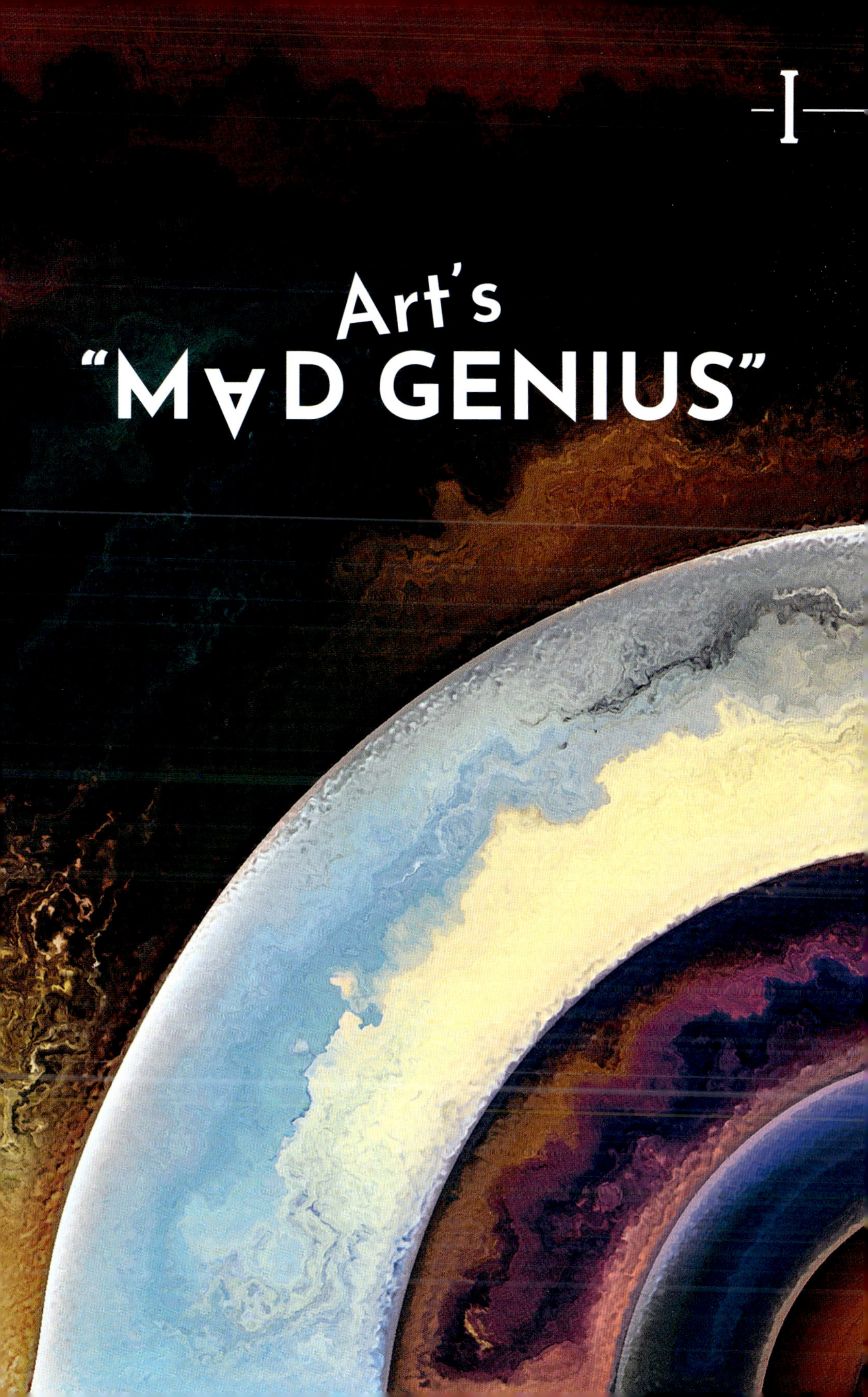
I
Art's
"MAD GENIUS"

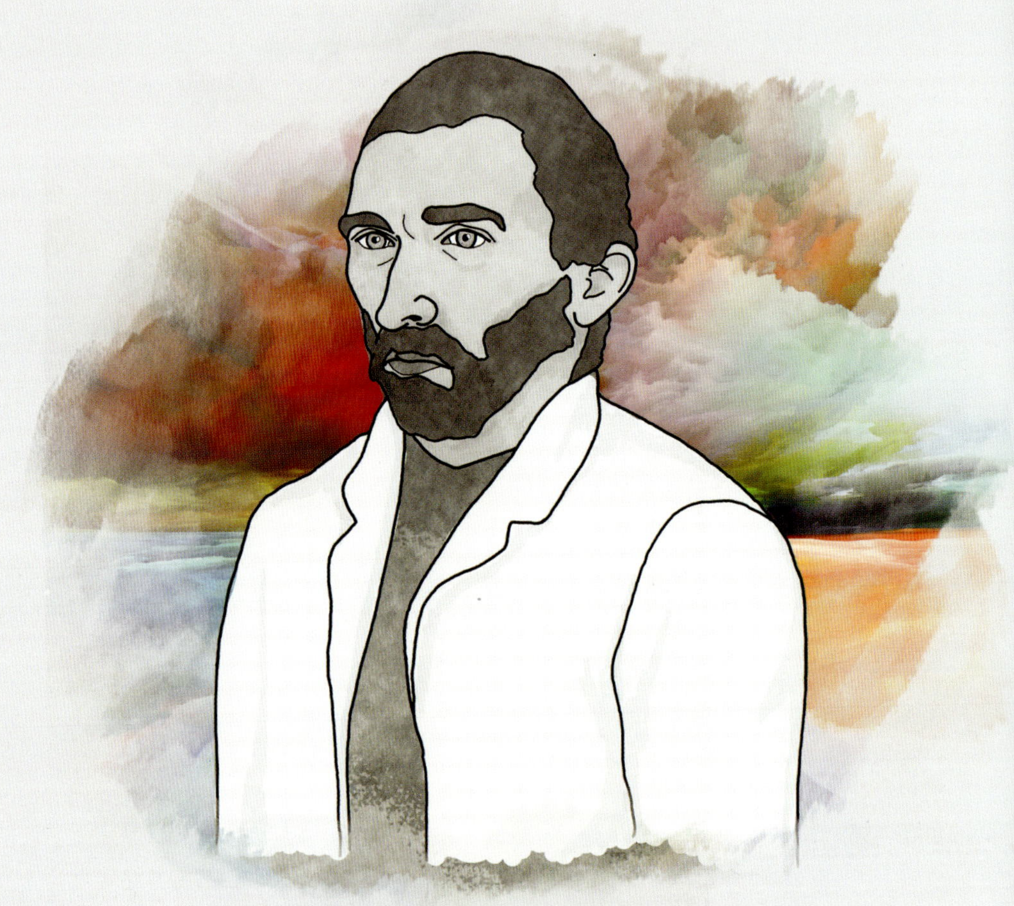

Vincent van Gogh

(March 30, 1853–July 29, 1890)

The heart of man is very much like the sea; it has its storms, it has its tides and in its depths it has its pearls too.

–VINCENT VAN GOGH[1]

If ever there was an artist who fascinated art historians and mental health professionals to the same degree, it is Vincent van Gogh. He has been the subject of countless art-historical surveys, and more than 150 doctors have attempted to diagnose him posthumously.[2] Throughout the rest of this book, we will provide you with an artist's biographical story and their related artworks in detail, with an eye toward the relationship between mental health and creativity. But van Gogh's story has been told through this lens countless times. It has inspired fiction and nonfiction books for all ages, as well as films and even song lyrics. Many of these stories go into great detail about his mental health. Therefore, instead of trying to encapsulate that story here, let's look instead at this cultural phenomenon: **How did van Gogh come to epitomize and exemplify the idea of "madness and genius" among artists?**

First, we acknowledge that the "fine line between madness and genius" has fascinated people for thousands of years. Dean Keith Simonton, writing for the *Psychiatric Times*, notes the link potentially dates back to the time of Aristotle.[3] The philosopher is quoted as saying, "No great mind has ever existed without a touch of madness."[4] Researchers across a multitude of disciplines have tried to figure out what the relationship is between insanity, mental health, and psychosis, on the one hand, and intelligence, innovation, and creativity on the other. While there are some who conclude there is no relationship, and others who believe the two are inextricable, most professionals fall somewhere in the middle. Even if we agree that such a relationship exists, to what extent, how, and why is still largely a mystery.

Simonton argues that "creativity and psychopathology are intimately connected," but that doesn't make "genius and madness tantamount to the same thing."[5] His view is that people with stabler mental health may tend toward less creative achievements, but that "outright psychopathology usually inhibits rather than helps creative expression."[6] Moreover, since plenty of artists don't exhibit signs of mental illness, you certainly can have one without the other. He concludes that there's a creativity cluster: that being creative requires some degree of dreaming "out of the box," which thus requires "defocused attention, divergent thinking, openness to experience, independence and nonconformity."[7] Some of these traits also correlate with psychopathology; however, when someone struggles too much with mental illness, it can negatively affect their creativity. Some argue that a creative impulse is actually more often a sign of mental health than "mental illness."[8] But, as we have discussed, there is no clear line between the two; a person may simply exist somewhere on the spectrum of "healthy" and "ill," and so there's a balance to be struck.

Perhaps van Gogh has so captured the imagination of those trying to understand this balance because he teetered along this line. His artwork represents times in his life of both relative wellness and so-called insanity. His paintings of nature continue to inspire the imagination of viewers today, but he also endeavored to paint what he saw, and not all of his life was spent soaking in the beauty of the sunbaked meadows of southern France. For instance, he spent one terrible year of his life in the Saint-Paul de Mausole asylum. His impression of the empty, seemingly endless hallways of the institution is represented in the decidedly bleak work *Corridor in the Asylum*.

We are also lucky to have many letters that give us a wealth of insight into van Gogh's creativity and state of mind. In fact, one diagnosis attributed to him posthumously is hypergraphia, a compulsion to write prolifically, which can be a symptom of both mania and epilepsy.[9] His letters from his year in the asylum indicate that life there was anything but pleasant. He wrote of his experience, "One continually hears shouts and terrible howls as of animals in a menagerie."[10] The terrifying sounds must have echoed horribly in that empty corridor. One patient he shared space with had auditory hallucinations, and van Gogh wrote that he seemed to be responding aloud to sounds in the corridor that no one else could hear—a haunting thought.

For the most part, van Gogh endeavored to paint the pleasant landscapes he remembered from his life before the institution.

Whenever possible, he would sit in the asylum's gardens, painting the beauty outdoors instead of the dull and dreary interior. This arguably resulted in some of his best work, including *Starry Night*. And he did heal, at least enough to leave the asylum, but only to fall prey to alcoholism and depression again. Famously, he got into a dramatic argument with friend and fellow artist Paul Gauguin, leading him to cut off part of his own ear. He then took the severed ear to a local prostitute and gave it to her as a gift.[11] Eventually, van Gogh died of what was most likely suicide at the age of thirty-seven. Professionals differ in their views, but a majority agree that his modern diagnosis would probably be bipolar depression with complications from alcohol addiction, which may have been his attempt at self-medicating. There's a history of family illness that further suggests bipolar depression, since the disorder is often genetic. His brother Cornelius also died by suicide, and his other two siblings, Theo and Wilhelmina, both died in asylums.[12] This wealth of tangible evidence of his journey as both an artist and a person with mental health issues may explain his popularity in regard to the subject.

It's also true that his artwork itself reflects the wild drama of his personal life and his vivid imagination. He is an important figure in art history as a leader in postimpressionist painting, in large part because his art was so expressive, and his mental illness may have played a part in that. Author Jonathan Jones describes a still life painted after leaving the asylum, which includes a medical self-help book, a letter from his brother Theo, a pipe, and a bottle of absinthe: "The very idea that a collection of objects, painted with fiery brushstrokes in heightened luminous colours, with ridges of thick impasto in some places and bare canvas in others, can reveal the state of someone's soul was utterly new. Van Gogh was its originator."[13] He goes on to describe how van Gogh's *Self-Portrait with Bandaged Ear* directly influenced German expressionist Ludwig Kirchner's self-portrait of war wounds and shell shock (which we now call PTSD).[14] The expressionist movement also influenced Hans Prinzhorn, who, as we'll see at the end of this book, was a leading force in exploring the creative impulses of people diagnosed with schizophrenia.[15]

Van Gogh's personal dramas inevitably lead to a question: How can someone who is suffering so much also find the will, energy, and talent to create such a beautiful and influential body of work? Yale professor Craig Wright, PhD, posits:

> Was van Gogh's "crazy" art the product of a tortured mental state . . . or a wholly lucid theory of art? Many of the distinctive qualities of van Gogh's style—his shimmering images, choice of color palette, and swirling two-color textures—were explained as artistic theory in letters to brother Theo, long before Vincent's mental disintegration. Van Gogh was well aware of the line between sanity and insanity, and he knew when he was sane and when he was not.[16]

Wright goes on to quote relevant letters from van Gogh to his brother. In 1882: "As a patient, you are not free to work as one should, and not up to it either," and, the following year: "Work is the only remedy. . . . If that does not help, one breaks down."[17] In another he writes, "I am so angry with myself because I cannot do what I should like to do, and at such a moment one feels as if one were lying bound hand and foot at the bottom of a deep, dark well, utterly helpless."[18] Van Gogh expressed in letters that around the time he was painting *Sunflowers*, just before Gauguin's visit and the ear-slicing incident, he was in one of his most prolific, important periods of creativity.[19] As Jones writes, "All this bold experiment, which van Gogh knew was unprecedented and a different way of seeing, was done at huge risk to his health and sanity."[20]

In other words, van Gogh knew that he struggled with symptoms of mental health issues and that art was the only thing that helped him feel better. And yet, at times—whether because of symptoms or his institutionalization—he was not able to use art in a therapeutic way. Perhaps it was mania that led to the amazing period of innovative productivity that he describes, but which also culminated in further damage to his sanity. When did art help van Gogh heal? Did his commitment to his art (and the ensuing financial struggles) contribute to his mental deterioration? Van Gogh experienced auditory and visual hallucinations, which he may have painted directly from.[21] If he never experienced those symptoms, would we have the swirling, dreamlike sky of *Starry Night*?

More than anything, van Gogh's prolific creativity during a life cut short may be what has inspired so many to draw him into this conversation. As psychiatrist Dietrich Blumer, MD, writes, "Vincent van Gogh's life has become a legend. Within the short span of 10 years, he persevered to overcome many struggles and failures to accomplish, through often feverish but always disciplined efforts, his goal to create exceptional works of art for the people."[22] All artists struggle with self-doubt, life-work balance, failure, and creative blocks. To look at what van Gogh was able to give the world, in spite of all of his challenges, is inspirational. Maybe that's why we still talk about him in this context, more than a century after his death.

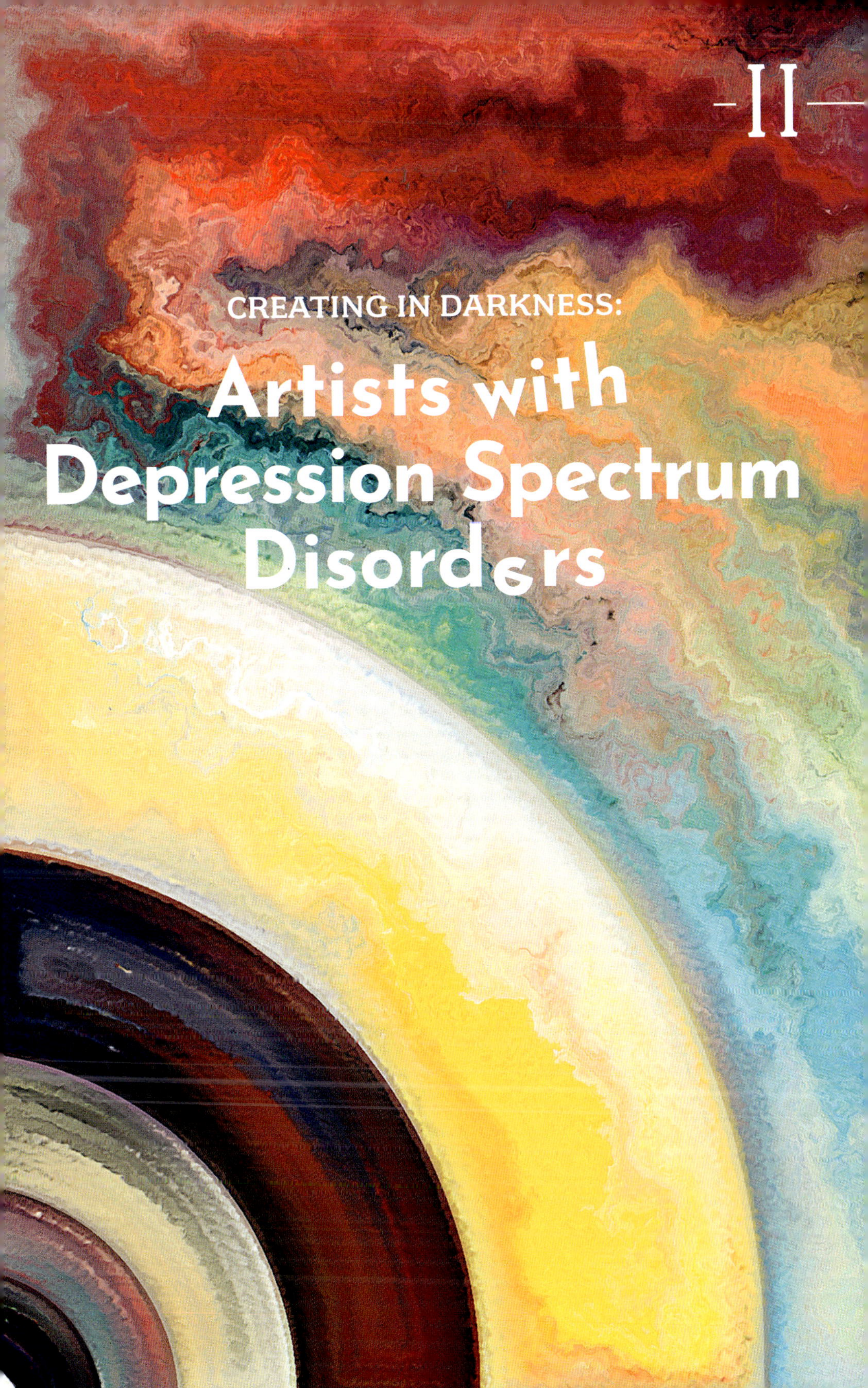

II

CREATING IN DARKNESS:

Artists with Depression Spectrum Disorders

With each passing decade, we learn more about mental health. It was not too long ago that people believed depression and bipolar disorder were two different things. Today, much of the professional psychiatric world believes that these two issues exist on a spectrum.

We are also increasingly aware that depression spectrum disorders affect a huge percentage of the population. **According to the National Institute for Mental Health, more than one-fifth of adults in the United States experience a mood disorder at some point in their lives.**[1] This is without considering people who experience symptoms of depression, but whose issues never rise to the level of diagnosis.

Since the experience of depression spectrum symptoms is so common, it's no surprise that a large percentage of artists fall somewhere on this spectrum as well. So, let's look at artists who are known or believed to have lived with major depression, bipolar depression, cyclothymia, and other related depression spectrum disorders.

UNDERSTANDING THE DEPRESSION SPECTRUM

Everyone who goes through a period of depression has their own unique experience. However, we can see enough similarities to identify the common types of depression. At one end of the spectrum is **major depression**. This is the classic picture of depression that may come to mind when you hear the word. It's the "totally fatigued, stay-in-bed, have trouble functioning and focusing, feel hopeless and worthless" kind of depression. At the other end of the spectrum is **bipolar**

depression (previously called manic depression). The difference between bipolar and major depression is that bipolar depression includes periods of mania or energetic highs that may cause restlessness, recklessness, and impulsivity. In between are various gradations, including hypomania, which tends to be a "lighter" version of mania with more-manageable symptoms. Another example is cyclothymia, which has the same "highs" and "lows" seen in bipolar disorder, but with cycles that last significantly longer. Postpartum depression and seasonal affective disorder (SAD) are other examples of common mood disorders on the depression spectrum.

Artists living with bipolar depression experience the energetic highs of mania or hypomania, which can be fertile times for making art. In contrast, creating art might seem impossible to artists with major depression, of which one key symptom is anhedonia, the loss of pleasure and interest in activities that once brought you joy. If you do get the urge to create, chances are that fatigue will sap that desire. How can someone make art when they don't even have the energy to make breakfast? Even the healthiest artists battle with self-esteem issues—how can people with depression get past it? It's an astounding feat that so many artists manage to create amazing art in spite of their battles with depression, rising out of the fog just long enough to put something incredible onto the page or canvas.

What is most important to consider is how the following artists' creativity and mental health issues are related, regardless of how their symptoms were labeled. **Did symptoms of depression help the artist create? Had their symptoms been better treated, would they have created more, or differently? Did the act of making art help them cope? Or did their relationship with their own artistic process (which, let's face it, can be fraught with fear and frustration for any person) worsen their depression?** The answer is different for every artist, and we can't answer for them. We can however keep these questions in mind as we delve into these artists' stories and, we hope, come to a more complete understanding of the relationship between depression and creativity.

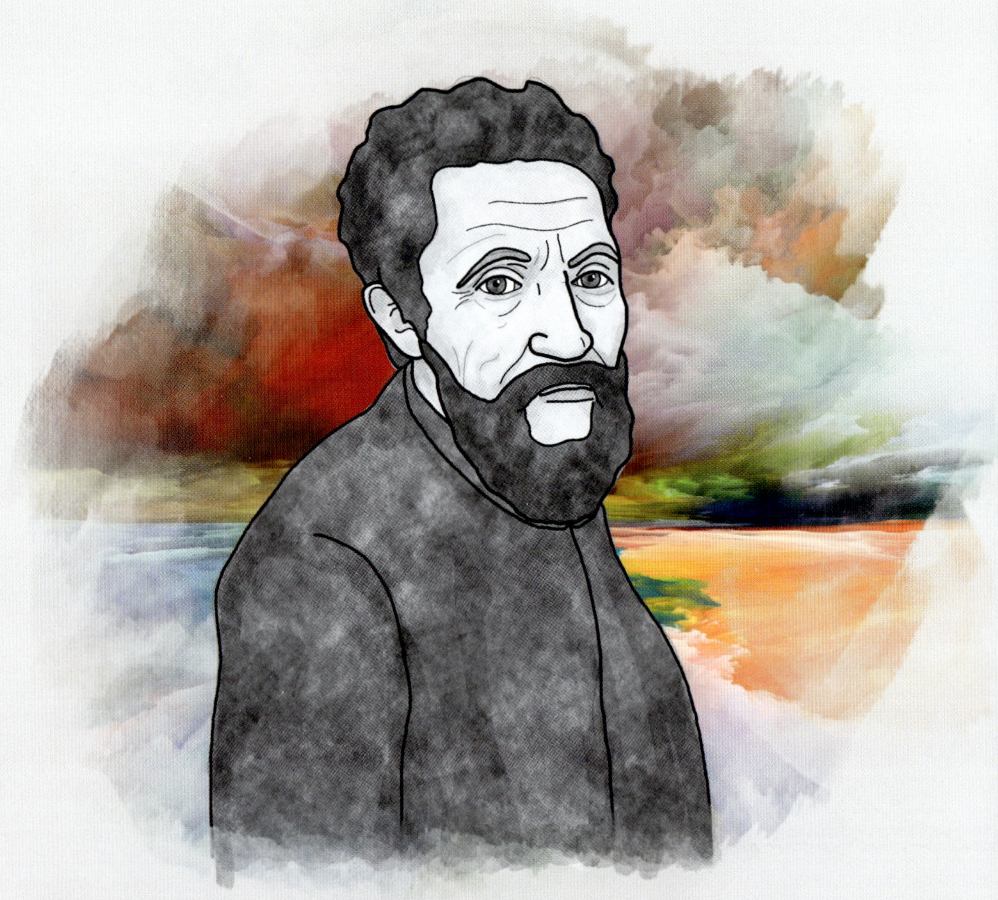

Michelangelo Buonarroti

(March 6, 1475–February 18, 1564)

I saw the angel in the marble and carved until I set him free.

–MICHELANGELO[1]

From the devastated grief emanating from the Virgin Mary cradling Christ in the *Pieta*, to the determined focus of *David* looking off into the distance before slaying Goliath, Michelangelo was a masterful sculptor of human emotion. And it is possible that this ability to channel and reflect our deepest feelings was related to his own struggles with depression. Though Michelangelo lived so long ago that it would be impossible to give him an accurate diagnosis, there is enough written about him, and by him, that historians, artists, and doctors have attempted to retroactively assess his mental health. Diagnoses have included everything from chronic kidney failure to autism spectrum disorder, but most professionals conclude that Michelangelo was a person experiencing depression. Art historian Jane Kromm writes, "The experiences of Michelangelo that may be construed as evidence of melancholia seem to cluster around several characteristic features. These are a sense of suffering from the harshness of existence, sadness revealed through introspective insight, grief and mourning, love, depression, and ruminative or obsessional concerns."[2]

Like all mental health issues, depression has biopsychosocial roots. In other words, it's the combination of nature and nurture. Our brain chemistry, our genetics, and our environment all are contributing factors that can cause depression to manifest, and dictate how. Neurochemical studies are in their infancy even today, so we cannot know anything specific about Michelangelo's brain chemistry. But we do know that both his surroundings and some of the trauma he experienced could have triggered a predisposition to. For example, we know that Michelangelo was only six years old when his mother passed away. He didn't know her well because his family had followed the practice of the time and had a wet nurse raise him away from home for most of the first three years of his life.[3] As one might imagine, he was emotionally attached to this caretaker. Her father and husband were stonecutters, and Michelangelo even said that he got his sculptural skills while nursing from her.[4] We can only speculate how devastating it was to be taken from her at age three and sent back to his parents, only to lose his mother a few years later.

Today, we know a lot about the role that early **childhood attachment** plays in mental health and in the formation of adult relationships. Attachment theory was developed by psychiatrist John Bowlby and further developed by psychologist Mary Ainsworth in the 1960s and '70s and has continued to evolve. It's a comprehensive field with many complex factors, but **the main idea is that the relationship we have with our earliest primary caregiver sets the blueprint for how we react in all future relationships**. The ideal is that your caregiver meets all your needs but also allows you to become self-sufficient, and thus you end up an emotionally healthy adult with a secure attachment style.

Many people, however, have one of the three forms of insecure attachment: **anxious, avoidant, or ambivalent**. The simplified explanation is that children whose needs aren't met become anxious or needy; children who grew up around rage, hostility, or trauma become avoidant in relationships and have trouble attaching to others; and children who got mixed messages become ambivalent and are often confused about what they want in relationships. What kind of attachment messages did Michelangelo receive when his family entrusted his care to a wet nurse who returned him at age three to a mother who died only three years later? It must have been complicated, to say the least.

Despite these early and likely confusing losses, Michelangelo thrived during his life in many ways. He began his art career young and showed much promise. Although his father wished for him to pursue a more professional career, he insisted on being an artist, first apprenticing under Ghirlandaio to learn fresco painting and then securing a job as a sculptor with the Medici family by the time he was fifteen.

Yet, although his career flourished, Michelangelo struggled emotionally from a very young age, finding the areas of love and sexuality to be particularly problematic. This could be related to the attachment issues described above, but he also likely battled internally with guilt and shame about homosexual feelings, which were considered extremely sinful in the Catholic society of Renaissance-era Italy.[5] Mostly undiscussed in his lifetime, Michelangelo's sexual orientation is up for debate, but it's been widely argued that he was a gay man struggling with religious concerns about his desires. Did these feelings perhaps come out in his art? Once societal views toward homosexuality began to progress, art historians focused extensively on the artist's passion for the male form and have suggested there are coded clues to his sexuality in his work.

Understanding Michelangelo's sexuality is complicated. Often his writings point to total abstinence or even repulsion by sex. Michelangelo seemed indifferent to women, and it's unknown whether he ever had sex in his lifetime. The only indication of any sort of passionate relationship is with Tommaso de' Cavalieri, who was "a young Roman nobleman for whom he developed a powerful infatuation."[6] Michelangelo was in his late fifties, de' Cavalieri in his early twenties, and Michelangelo wrote him hundreds of letters and poems expressing his love.[7] This relationship was long ignored in scholarly study of the artist due to the censorship of the poems by his nephew, Michelangelo the Younger, who published many of them posthumously but changed the pronouns to make the verses heterosexual.[8] When this came to light, historians debated whether this was simply platonic brotherly love or a more passionate love. Perhaps even Michelangelo wasn't sure.

Michelangelo's sexuality could not have been an easy situation to navigate given the time in which he lived. Toward the end of his long life, he collaborated with a pupil to write his biography, in which he carefully alludes to the situation, explaining how at the end of the fifteenth century, when Michelangelo was a teenager coming into his own sexuality, there existed much tension between two competing viewpoints: the Platonic Academy's faithful followers, who believed in the beauty of the male body (particularly young male bodies, as influenced by the Greek), and the followers of Dominican friar Girolamo Savonaro, who campaigned against nudity and "sodomites."[9] Michelangelo struggled to reconcile his aesthetic appreciation of the male body and the idea of sexuality and nudity as Catholic sins.[10]

This attempt to reconcile two very different belief systems, as well as pressing, immediate stressors related to his work, may have combined with a genetic predisposition to depression and contributed to major depressive periods for Michelangelo. **Though creating art may have been cathartic, the professional pressures of the job were often difficult to handle.** He often took much longer than necessary to complete his works, sometimes not finishing them at all. This seems to have been, at least at times, a direct result of the lethargy and self-doubt that come with depression, and a cycle in which the unfinished work leads to further ruminating thoughts that exacerbate the issue. As an example, let's consider Michelangelo's Florentine *Pieta* (different from the *Pieta* we previously mentioned). He worked on the sculpture for eight years and, in the words of one biographer, "poured his depression over his life into the statue."[11] Depression can feel ugly, and whether or not the work was objectively reflecting that, Michelangelo finally got so frustrated with what he perceived as the dismal results of his labor that he attempted to destroy the sculpture with a chisel. Historians believe he carved his own likeness as Saint Nicodemus in the composition, which begs the question of whether he was attacking a part of himself when he attacked the statue.[12]

Michelangelo may be best recognized for painting the ceiling of the Sistine Chapel, but the world is lucky he managed to complete the magnificent mural at all. Letters indicate that he dragged through the work in a state of exhaustion and depression.[13] It probably didn't help matters that the artist didn't enjoy painting; he considered himself a sculptor and took painting commissions only in order to pay the bills.[14] **Many working artists will recognize this struggle to find a balance between working creatively and working for financial stability, and artists who struggle with mental health issues may find this balance particularly precarious.** Biographer Martin Gayford notes that, in times of deep depression, Michelangelo would often give in to fatigue and opt not to work on projects that didn't add positively to his life, even if it meant giving up money. Other times, he would feel compelled to take on unwanted jobs even though they exacerbated his depression.[15]

Michelangelo started the Sistine Chapel in 1508. By 1512, Pope Julius, afraid he wouldn't see the ceiling painted before his own death, pestered the artist almost daily for updates on its progress, but to no avail.[16] Michelangelo complained to the pope, often describing physical ailments that may or may not have been symptoms of his mental state. **Depression often manifests in physical illness**: headaches, gastrointestinal distress, fatigue, insomnia, and body aches are common examples. Michelangelo, despite being a strong, healthy, thirty-three-year-old man when he started the project, "complained of aches, discomfort, tired bones, and feeling old."[17] And it's been widely documented in biographies about him that he had difficulties or eccentricities around both his eating and sleeping habits, which could also be possible symptoms of depression.[18] Michelangelo would have continued trying to perfect the painting if the pope hadn't said, "Enough is enough," and declared it done.[19] Ironically, the Sistine ceiling is one of his most famous works, and yet he seemingly detested every minute of its creation.

Although Michelangelo is best known for his work in the visual arts, he was also a prolific poet. One of his poems, the unfinished canzone, laments the sadness of time lost. Some believe that the poem is in response to three years he felt he wasted creating the facade of the Basilica of San Lorenzo.[20] The poem begins:

> What's to become of me?
> What's this you're doing
> to my charred old heart you've made such ashes of?
> Suppose you tell me, Love,
> so I'll know how it stands with me, what trouble's brewing.

And goes on later to say:

> No ordeal lasts when age begins to tell.
> That's why I seem like ice the flames enwrap:
> It shrinks, writhes to escape, but won't invite.
> I'm old. My sole defense is death, whose might
> Can ward off your brutal arm, your barbs that rain
> Their piercing pain on pain.[21]

The artist also left hints regarding his mental state in his written correspondence. He once wrote to an artist friend that he was unable to work due to "*mal sano*," a phrase that could mean poor physical or mental health.[22] Other times he explicitly names his depression, as in this 1525 letter: "Several other gentlemen kindly invited me to go and have supper with them, which gave me the greatest pleasure, as I emerged a little from my depression, or rather from my obsession. I not only enjoyed the supper, which was extremely pleasant, but also, and even more than this, the discussions which took place."[23]

From what we can surmise, Michelangelo appears to be a quintessential example of an artist who created great works in the face of depression, and in some instances it seems the work itself reflects his struggles. **Without the unique ways in which his brain worked, including the depressive periods he endured, would he have created works that touch so deeply on these universal aspects of human emotion?** Yet, might he have accomplished even more if depression hadn't been holding him back? What masterpieces could he have given the world without the exhaustion and self-flagellation that came with a depressed mind?

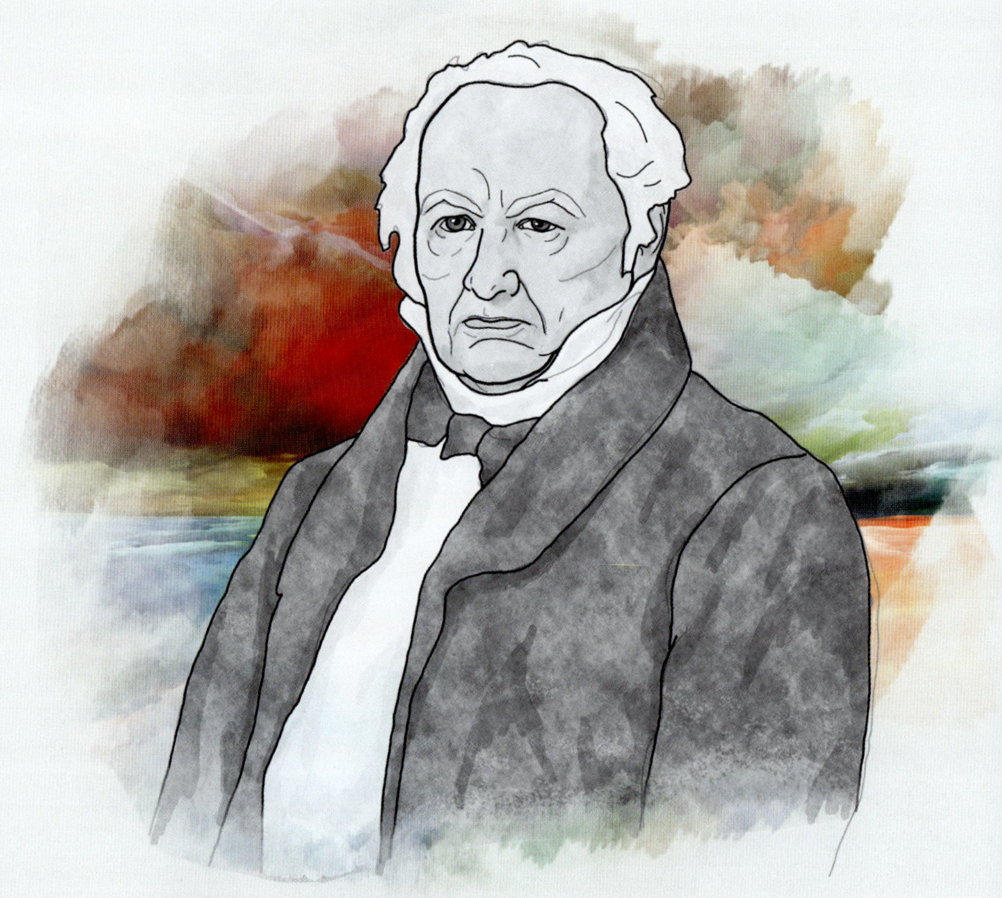

Francisco Goya

(March 30, 1746–April 16, 1828)

Fantasy, abandoned by reason, produces impossible monsters; united with it, she is the mother of the arts and the origin of marvels.

—FRANCISCO GOYA[1]

Art history has categorized Francisco Goya's work into two periods: the light and happy early art, and the later work filled with monsters and ugliness.[2] **Many suggest it was Goya's depression, which coincided with a variety of physical ailments, that caused his artwork's progression into darkness.** Of course, since he was diagnosed in the eighteenth century, it's difficult to pinpoint exactly what Goya was suffering from. Most believe that his mental health issues were a symptom of either syphilis or of antisyphilis treatment. Syphilis has been known to cause a variety of psychiatric conditions, including depression, mania, psychosis, and changes in personality.[3] Goya himself experienced hallucinations. He also had other chronic illnesses, including eventual deafness, which can cause or coincide with depression.[4] Authors Felisati and Sperati write, "The increasing severity of his deafness, as often occurs, would have played a not indifferent role in inducing the sense of melancholy, isolation, seeking refuge in fantasy."[5] There's also evidence to suggest a genetic history of mental illness, since Goya had an aunt and uncle who suffered from "insanity."[6] Plus, there was the not-so-insignificant fact that he worked with a lot of lead-based paint, which could have impacted both his physical and mental health. Researcher Laura L. Casey reviewed all of the likely medical or environmental causes for his symptoms and concluded that the most likely diagnosis is "somatic manifestation of severe depression."[7] In other words, she argues that **depression wasn't simply a symptom but was in fact the underlying illness.**

While Goya's various illnesses and genetic predisposition may suggest a biochemical cause for his depression, we cannot discount the emotional impact of his life experience as a contributing factor. Traumatic circumstances, as we'll explore later in this book, often cause or exacerbate mental health conditions. For instance, grief can often mutate into depression. Goya had an unhappy marriage, complicated by the fact that the couple had several pregnancies that ended in miscarriage, and children who died very young.[8] In fact, only one of their children survived into adulthood. Some have posited that Goya passed syphilis on to his wife and that the disease may have been a root cause of the miscarriages and deaths in infancy. In a 2006 article published in the *International Journal of Surgery*, Laura L. Casey writes, "It has often been suggested that Goya's depiction of Saturn gorging himself upon one of his progenies is illustrative of the artist's own sense of guilt and self-loathing resulting from what he may, quite naturally, have perceived to be a degree of personal responsibility for the untimely deaths of his children."[9]

Regardless of the root cause of his depression, we know that Goya went through at least two, and possibly four, specific periods of extreme illness, during which he also showed symptoms of major depression. In one instance, the doctors diagnosed "delirium" caused by typhoid fever. Delirium's symptoms include trouble concentrating, disorganized speech, sleep troubles, psychomotor changes, and memory difficulties, which could also be symptoms of depression.[10] **Goya also tended to isolate himself, which worsened his condition. This solitude freed him to immerse himself in a fantasy life, which was what made his later work so emotionally evocative, but it was likely no help to his mental health.** Unfortunately, people with depression tend to self-isolate due to a combination of symptoms including low self-esteem, irritability, and fatigue. However, isolation and loneliness have been proven to have adverse health consequences, including causing or exacerbating depression.[11]

At age fifty, Goya started the series *Los Caprichos*. The illustration from this series titled *The Sleep of Reason Produces Monsters* (*El sueño de la razón produce monstruos*) is arguably one of the best visual representations of his battle with mental illness. It is filled with darkness and monsters of the night, anxiety and suffering reflected in images of a black cat, bats, and other strange creatures surrounding the dreaming figure. Laura Casey describes the sleeping person as "consumed by despair and haunted by a writhing mass of nightmarish forms unwittingly conjured by his own addled mind."[12] Peter Klein writes that "according to Goya's idea, the imagination is not only the mother of the arts—his own art included—but in the end also the origin of madness." In other words, imagination is inextricably linked to both the creation of great art and the devastation of mental illness, and Goya believed that his creativity and his "madness" derived from the same place. To him, his ability to create masterful work may not have been possible without the depression and hallucinations he endured.

Felisati and Serati go on to express how the darkness seen in *Los Caprichos* only grew in Goya's later work, best reflected in the "Black Paintings," the most famous of which is *Saturn Devouring His Son*. To the authors this work reflects the anguish Goya felt at the end of his life: "Dominating were wide-open mouths and the whites of eye-sockets; the figures, monstrous and tragic, expressing all the desperation of the author." Casey reminds us that although this piece was created late in his life, it might reference an earlier time; remember her suggestion that Saturn represents Goya's complicated grief and guilt from losing so many of his children.

Goya's work isn't just representative of his own illness. He was fascinated with "madness" and painted numerous images of people living in mental asylums after visiting these institutions and seeing the horrors there. Not one to sugarcoat things with a pretty name, Goya aptly called one of his most famous paintings on this subject *The Madhouse*, and in it we see the chaos of the asylum. Naked men grapple with each other and with invisible foes in a desolate courtyard. Chiefs and kings represent authority figures that suggest the troubling power dynamics in eighteenth-century asylums. Goya's interest in these madhouses and engrained belief that his own so-called madness inspired his creativity reflects an interesting duality in how mental health was perceived during Goya's lifetime. As Peter Klein explains:

> Towards the end of the eighteenth century, there was a growing interest in and even fascination with manifestations of insanity and its relationship with reason, nature and society. Basically, there were two different approaches. On the one hand, contemporary medicine considered madness in a rationalistic, enlightened and increasingly scientific way, starting to isolate lunatics as potentially curable patients in special institutions and attempting empirically to classify the various mental

> diseases. On the other hand, there was a more ambiguous, partly romanticising and idealising, attitude in literature, philosophy and art, which placed madness next to genius, as a source of creativity and as an opportunity for a deeper, more genuine and non-alienated experience of human life.[13]

Goya's art can be best understood when keeping these coexisting cultural attitudes in mind. **His work is the reflection of a man searching for answers about the human condition—pain, grief, torment—both within himself and in society.** At the same time, the darkness is where he finds inspiration, his own creative impulse driven by this angst and misery.

To this end, we cannot ignore the political climate that influenced Goya's life and artwork. Goya lived during the Enlightenment, a period of history that brought political, social, and economic changes to Europe by emphasizing science, rational thinking, questioning of government (particularly monarchies), and separation of church and state. However, in 1808, France invaded Spain and the new monarch, Ferdinand VII, did away with much of the progress made during the Spanish Enlightenment. Spanish citizens were executed en masse. At this time, Goya began documenting the violence, criticizing the events in a series of prints titled *The Disasters of War*.[14] As we will see in future chapters on trauma, particularly when we look at Gustave Doré, war can have a huge impact on an individual's mental health. We can't know for sure how the wartime experience effected Goya, but with close to one hundred works of art depicting this time in his life, it must have left an indelible impression upon his psyche.

Disability & Illness

As we see with Francisco Goya and Frida Kahlo, living with a disability or serious illness can directly negatively impact one's mental health (especially the farther back in history you look, as much progress has been made in the realm of disability rights in recent years). It's logical that when there is a drastic or traumatic change to one's body, one's sense of self may become warped, and studies have shown that living with a disability is correlated to a higher risk of depression.[1] Creative pursuits can help people work through this type of ongoing trauma.[2] For example, photographer Jo Spence chronicled her battle with breast cancer on film in order to confront her illness and regain a sense of empowerment over her body. Spence then developed this body of work into a therapeutic model of healing called 'photo-therapy,' taking pictures of other people working through personal trauma.

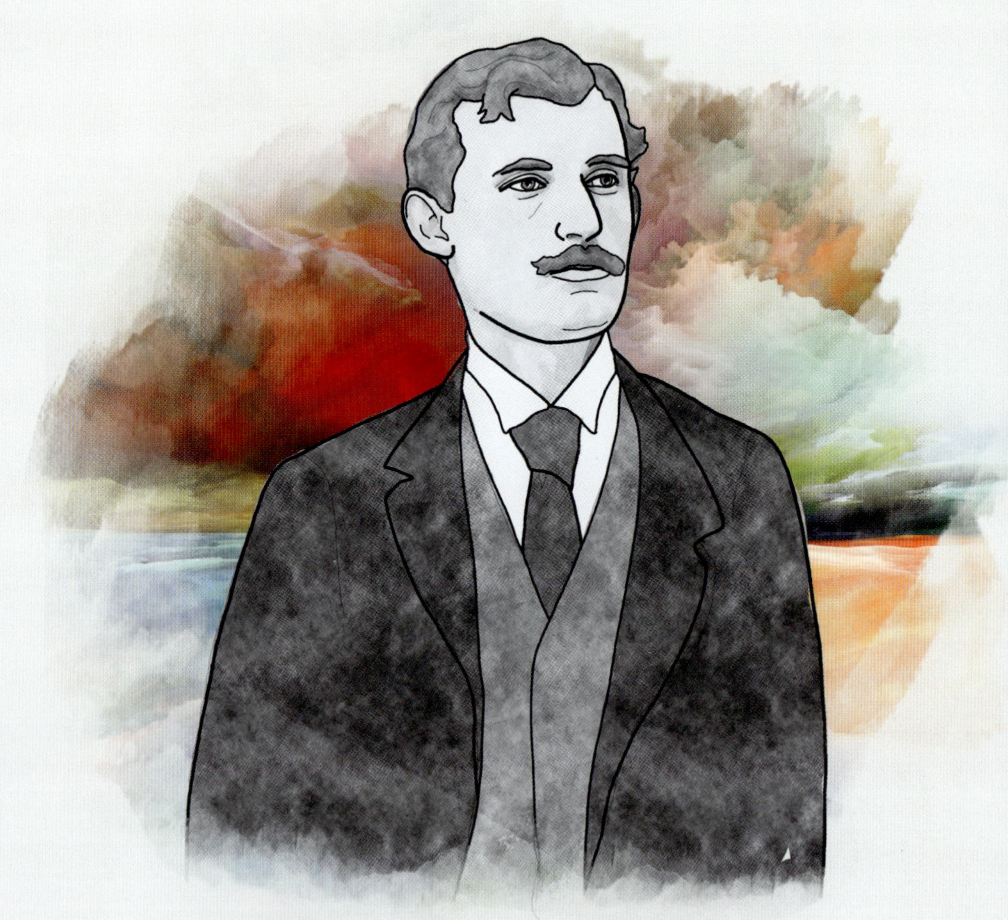

Edvard Munch

(December 12, 1863–January 23, 1944)

My sufferings are part of my self and my art. They are indistinguishable from me, and their destruction would destroy my art. I want to keep those sufferings.

–EDVARD MUNCH[1]

Even people who don't know much about art will probably recognize Edvard Munch's *The Scream*. The iconic 1893 painting is part of a narrative series called *Frieze of Life* that was first shown in 1902 at an exhibition of the Berlin Secession art movement. *The Scream* ended the set, which began with a painting titled *Anxiety* (1894). Biographer Sue Prideaux calls the five "anxiety" paintings in the twenty-two-work series (including *The Scream)* "the most internalized section of the narrative" and says that they describe "every form of anxiety that affects the individual; from the intrinsic self-doubt present in every soul at its conception, to guilt conscience . . . to the self-doubt of the artistic crucified by the critics ... to the final breaking point."[2] **It is clear from these emotion-filled paintings that Munch was intimately familiar with anxiety, which was, in his case, most likely a symptom of bipolar disorder.**

The Scream is such a vivid, dramatic painting that it's unsurprisingly sparked many interpretations over the years. One reading of the work is that it provides an accurate picture of what it's like to live inside the bipolar brain at the height of mania. Some people mistakenly assume that mania is a pleasant or exhilarating state for people with bipolar disorder. From the outside it can look exciting, productive, and creative in comparison to the lows of depression. It is true that these positive feelings manifest at times, particularly when someone is experiencing **hypomania**, which has symptoms that are similar to mania but not so intense as to rise to a manic diagnosis. For example, people may experience delusions of grandeur in which they think that they are capable of creating amazing work, which is creatively inspiring. In a manic state, in contrast, they might actually believe that they are the most powerful artist on the planet, receiving their gifts from the universe, and that everything they create is the best thing that has ever been created.

At some point, though, the rush of the "high" gets to be too much, and both the body and mind get overstimulated. This can lead to an inability to process one's surroundings to a point that is overwhelming, and the individual may experience paranoia, panic, or delusions, often from lack of sleep. Authors Demitri and Janice Papolos, writing about bipolar depression, suggest that *The Scream* is one of the best visual artistic representations of this experience.[3] On the basis of Munch's own diary descriptions, *The Scream* does seem to have developed from a hallucination or panic attack It was, for him, the representation of "a moment of existential crisis" that happened during what was otherwise a normal day. While walking with friends, the sky suddenly began to appear as if it were bleeding, giving him an intense anxious and claustrophobic feeling, as though he was watching nature itself scream through the clouds.[4]

To better understand Munch's state of mind, it is useful to know his family history, which was marked by a series of significant losses. When Munch was just five years old, his mother died. Less than a decade later, a favorite sister passed away. This trauma in particular was pivotal in his life, and, as we will come to see, he painted and repainted images of his sister over the years. Later, before he was thirty, he would lose a brother, a grandfather, and his father.[5] Munch had a fraught relationship with his father prior to his death. The man verbally abused Munch, even invoking Munch's dead mother, saying that she would not be proud of her children.[6] He vehemently disapproved of Munch's decision to be an artist, and tried to sway him from that vocation until the day he died (leaving the family impoverished and Munch to bear the financial burden).[7] Munch wrote that the man "was temperamentally nervous and obsessively religious—to the point of psychoneurosis," and that he felt that he had inherited his father's "madness."[8]

Edvard's sister Laura was diagnosed with mental illness and spent much of her life in an asylum, as Edvard would also eventually do. Laura was institutionalized at a time that was interesting in terms of the history of her illness, which was likely a schizoaffective disorder. In 1887, German physician Emile Kraeplin distinguished a set of symptoms that he called "dementia praecox."[9] This was the first time that a doctor differentiated this disorder from manic depression (today called bipolar depression). In 1911, Swiss psychiatrist Eugen Bleuler renamed the condition schizophrenia.[10] Schizoaffective disorder is essentially a combination of a mood disorder (depression or bipolar depression) and the psychosis of schizophrenia.[11]

The parallels between Laura's and Edvard's life were reflected in Munch's artwork. For example, biographer Sue Prideaux writes of *Self-Portrait with Wine Bottle*, a painting that shows a lonely old Munch sitting at a table surrounded by garish greens and reds, as "a picture of absolute isolation" and "extreme depression."[12] Prideaux calls *Self-Portrait with Wine Bottle* a "companion piece for *Melancholy (Laura)*, in which an isolated Laura sits at a table in the asylum.[13] The red, swirling tabletop is designed to look like a biopsy of her complicated brain."[14]

It is very common in families where one member is struggling for that person to receive the majority of the rest of the family's attention and focus. In family therapy this is called the **identified patient.** For example, if one person in the family is diagnosed with alcoholism, though everyone in the family has their own challenges, the alcoholic individual will be the center of attention, even if that attention is negative and more akin to blame. In Munch's family, it was Laura's mental health issues that took center stage. For much of his life, Munch would send large sums of money to care for Laura, covering expenses such as a private room in the asylum where she lived.[15] Although he suffered with his own mental health challenges, Munch felt financially responsible for his family and managed to work often enough to support them. With this family dynamic at play, a person can go a long time without identifying their own issues, focusing on the identified patient's problems instead.

Munch left college after just one year to pursue his career as a painter and worked prolifically for decades.[16] In much of his early art, he does seem to be working through his experiences with trauma and mental illness. Hina Azeem describes his early pieces as pessimistic, expressing—through both content and color—feelings of "death, anxiety, and depression."[17] Many of these paintings are directly autobiographical. For example, *The Sick Child* depicts Sophie, the sister who died when he was a young teenager, as very ill, just before her death. He painted it in 1885, and it was considered his first masterpiece.[18] Munch repainted images of Sophie in sickness again and again for the next thirty years, a repetition that suggests a continuing attempt to process that loss.[19] Sophie died of tuberculosis, an illness he also had as a child, which also killed their mother. Munch harbored guilt over Sophie's death, perhaps for surviving when she did not, and also feared that he was the one who infected her.[20] He re-created this image approximately every ten years, effectively marking the decades of his life.[21] Tied up with his feelings about Sophie's death may have been angst over the painting itself. When it debuted in 1886 in a central position at an exhibit, it was met with "outcries and laughter" and was "widely criticized and ridiculed."[22]

Aside from death, another recurring theme in Munch's work is the depiction of "a forlorn man and a domineering woman," which likely emerges from his passion for, and depression over losing, his first love, Millie Thaulow.[23] Their relationship lasted just two years but seemed to affect Munch greatly, since his work continued to depict troubled couples almost a decade after their separation. In 1894, he painted *Ashes*, in which a woman dressed to show a red slip beneath her white dress stares out at the viewer while her lover faces away and hangs his head in anguish. The woman reportedly looks much like the real-life Millie.[24] As with *The Sick Child*, Munch reworked this image repeatedly in various mediums. **Repetition of thoughts, or a "ruminating mind," is a symptom of anxiety and depression that may explain Munch's constant re-creating of traumatic life events in his art.** Of course, artists do make many versions of a piece before they consider it "done," so one could argue this was his creative process at play. But it's notable that the themes he repeated most were the events that were hardest for him in life, suggesting that making art was a way of processing the trauma, not simply an attempt to get the right color or composition.

In 1898, Munch met another woman, Tulla Larsen, and entered into a relationship that would also come to torment him.[25] In this case, however, it was not that Tulla rejected him but rather that she so aggressively pursued Munch that he felt compelled to respond even though he didn't return her affections. A telling painting from this time is *The Dance of Life*, in which a man dances with a woman who looks a lot like Millie, while a woman, representing Tulla, appears on either side of him, wearing white on one side and black on the other.[26] Painted just a year or so after they met, the image seems to represent his conflicted and unresolved feelings. In 1903, after a full year apart, he was told that Tulla was suicidally depressed and desperate to see him, so he went to visit her. The details are murky, but they got into an argument that resulted in Munch shooting off part of his finger.[27] Although the physical injury was minimal, Munch couldn't reconcile the event psychologically, blowing it up into a huge loss, made even more dramatic by the fact that Tulla married another man shortly after.[28] Munch re-created *The Dance of Life* multiple times over, as well, painting the scene as late as 1925, almost thirty years later.

In the summer of 1907, as his biographer Sue Prideaux describes, "Munch plunged into a frenziedly productive few months between June and September, when his health at last broke down totally and he had to be admitted to an asylum."[29] He had fought hospitalization for many years, knowing that he was suffering from mental illness but afraid that the treatment would negatively affect his art.[30] **This suggests that perhaps, like Goya, Munch believed that his depression and his creativity derived from the same source, and that without one, he could not have the other.** Bipolar depression is characterized in part by highs and lows, and living with this duality may make one feel that opposites must coexist.

Munch wanted to live without mental health treatment for as long as he could. However, throughout 1907 and into 1908 Munch began to experience paralysis and hallucinations. As a result, he ended up checking himself into Dr. Daniel Jacobson's nerve clinic, the Kornhaug Sanatorium, in Copenhagen, "which had a reputation for 'curing' artists." He was diagnosed with "*dementia paralytica* as a result of alcohol poisoning."[31] This gave Munch a dual diagnosis of alcohol misuse and what today would be called bipolar disorder with psychosis.[32] How does that differ from his sister Laura's schizoaffective disorder? Currently, the Diagnostic and Statistical Manual of Mental Disorders (DSM) would say that someone like Laura might have psychotic experiences even when not going through depression or mania, whereas someone like Edvard would have psychosis only as part of the manic state. Back then, Dr. Kraeplin worked hard to distinguish these different kinds of psychosis and separate schizophrenia out as its own condition. However, there is much overlap between these conditions, and diagnosticians increasingly wonder if they're all part of the same spectrum. In fact, bipolar depression with psychosis can convert into schizoaffective disorder over time.[33]

Regardless of diagnosis, we know that Munch struggled with symptoms of depression and psychosis and that he had suicidal thoughts.[34] In the asylum, Munch rested, took curative baths, received "a gentle application of weak electrical current," and was given "strong sleeping drops." As a result, both the paralysis and the auditory hallucinations began to wane.[35] And, despite what Munch had feared, his creativity did not diminish along with his symptoms. In fact, he was quite prolific during his time at the asylum, devising his own writing-and-painting cure.[36] **Instead of allowing the treatment for his mental illness to rob him of his creative impulse, he actively used art as a treatment.**

And it may have worked. In the asylum, Dr. Jacobson asked to be painted by the artist, and Munch did so, saying that he enjoyed the control he had painting his subject, a subject who, as the doctor, was usually in the position of authority. He said, "There was no weakness in my art; it was stronger than him. It had not been destroyed." The style of Munch's work changed by the time he was released. Although not necessarily optimistic, the themes and colors were not nearly as morose as they had once been.[37] *The Sun*, for example, is a huge departure from the anxiety-producing sunset in *The Scream*; this painting is brightly colored and seems to celebrate the joy of nature, rather than reflect fear or torment.[38]

Munch was in the asylum for less than a year. He reduced his drinking and his mental health seemingly improved, and he would go on to live another four decades. During the rest of his life, Munch spent much of his time alone in retreat at his estate, devoted to his own mental health. He wrote in 1920 that his life at this time was a battle just to stay afloat.[39] Though he continued to paint, most of his postasylum work has gone unrecognized, perhaps suggesting an overemphasis on his mental breakdown in interpretations of his art. He painted a lot of landscapes at his estate, but late in life he would return to old autobiographical themes, and also the illnesses of aging (such as *Self-Portrait with Afflicted Eye*). Karl Ove Knausgaard argues for the value in looking at the whole span of Munch's career as "a more than sixty[-]year[-]long continual search for meaning, a continual exploration of the world through painting, full of failure, fumbling and banality, but also of wildness, audacity and triumph."[40]

Let's return now, with our understanding of Munch's life experiences, to *The Scream*. *The Scream* has been widely reproduced on everything from coffee mugs to pillowcases, no doubt in large part because it represents a universal human emotion. Did Munch's depressive illness and hallucinations give him the insight necessary to capture this emotion in such a powerful way that it continues to impact people over a century after its creation? The painting was highly personal to Munch, who said he painted it "to represent his soul."[41] He ignored realism or perfectionism in favor of spilling his emotions onto the canvas in a way that was wholly original.[42]

The Scream we are all familiar with is not the only version in existence. Like so many of his works, Munch re-created this image over and over, and it took him almost two years of tweaking to arrive at the now-famous image. In the beginning, it wasn't a ghostlike screaming figure depicted, but instead showed a man in profile looking out over a bridge in front of the swirling clouds. Over time, the man's position changed; sometimes he had a hat, and sometimes he was closer to the bridge. Of course, in the final image, the man faces front, his face distorted in a scream of terror, right alongside the screaming sky. As Harvard professor of psychology Albert Rothenberg describes it, these changes reflect a healthful creative process in which Munch achieved catharsis through painting, allowing him to reflect the shared human experience of suffering, rather than simply recording his own hallucinatory episode.[43]

Although often left out of analyses of *The Scream*, historical context is also important to the understanding of Munch's work. Art historian Jon Mann suggests it is "illustrative of a host of late-19th-century concerns about the health of the human mind at a time when modern cities were rising, old power structures were being overturned, and the possibility of a great cataclysm (eventually realized in World War I) loomed large."[44] Individual human psychology is not inextricable from what is going on in the world around us, and the state of society at any given point in time will inevitably influence artists. Munch was an intellectual who was interested in human psychology and who understood the societal tumult of his time. All of these factors likely came into to play as he worked on *The Scream*, bringing his personal understanding of trauma and terror to the canvas in a way that speaks to our collective souls. It is a reminder both of our shared pain and of the gift of art to help us recognize common truths.

Influence on Contemporary Artists: Tracey Emin

Artists are always grappling with what came before, and when it comes to art that deals with issues of mental health the situation is no different. Many artists look to the past for inspiration, considering how their predecessors conveyed emotional turmoil, as well as reconsidering that historical visual language through a contemporary lens. Having created one of the most iconic images representing angst and anxiety in *The Scream*, Edvard Munch has predictably influenced many contemporary artists, including British feminist artist Tracey Emin.

Emin is famous for incorporating autobiographical themes of depression and trauma into her work, and has had a lifelong fascination with Edvard Munch, even going so far as to curate a 2021 exhibition of her own art alongside that of the Norwegian artist's at the Royal Academy of Arts in London, titled *Loneliness of the Soul*.[1] His influence on Emin is immediately apparent: both artists' work is deeply vulnerable, exposing their deepest, darkest secrets, fears, and miseries. Emin's seminal installation *My Bed*, for instance, conveys a setting that will be familiar to many who have experienced or encountered severe depression: a disheveled bed. With rumpled, sweat-stained sheets and a surrounding pile of trash, cigarette butts, and empty alcohol bottles, *My Bed* represents the aftermath of an episode of days-long suicidal depression. Beds are a recurring theme in Munch's work, as well, whether as the site of trauma in paintings of his dying sister's sickbed, or as a representation of deep loneliness in solemn paintings of solitary figures alone in their rooms.

Referencing Munch even more explicitly is Emin's *Homage to Edvard Munch and All My Dead Children*, a video piece performed outside Munch's seaside home, in which she gives voice to the wailing figure in *The Scream*, expressing the anguish of her experience with abortion.[2] We can see through these examples how Emin was inspired by Munch's expressions of pain, using similar strategies to express her personal turmoil. Like Munch, Emin's work resonates more universally as well and speaks to a broader human suffering—in her case, especially the suffering of women.

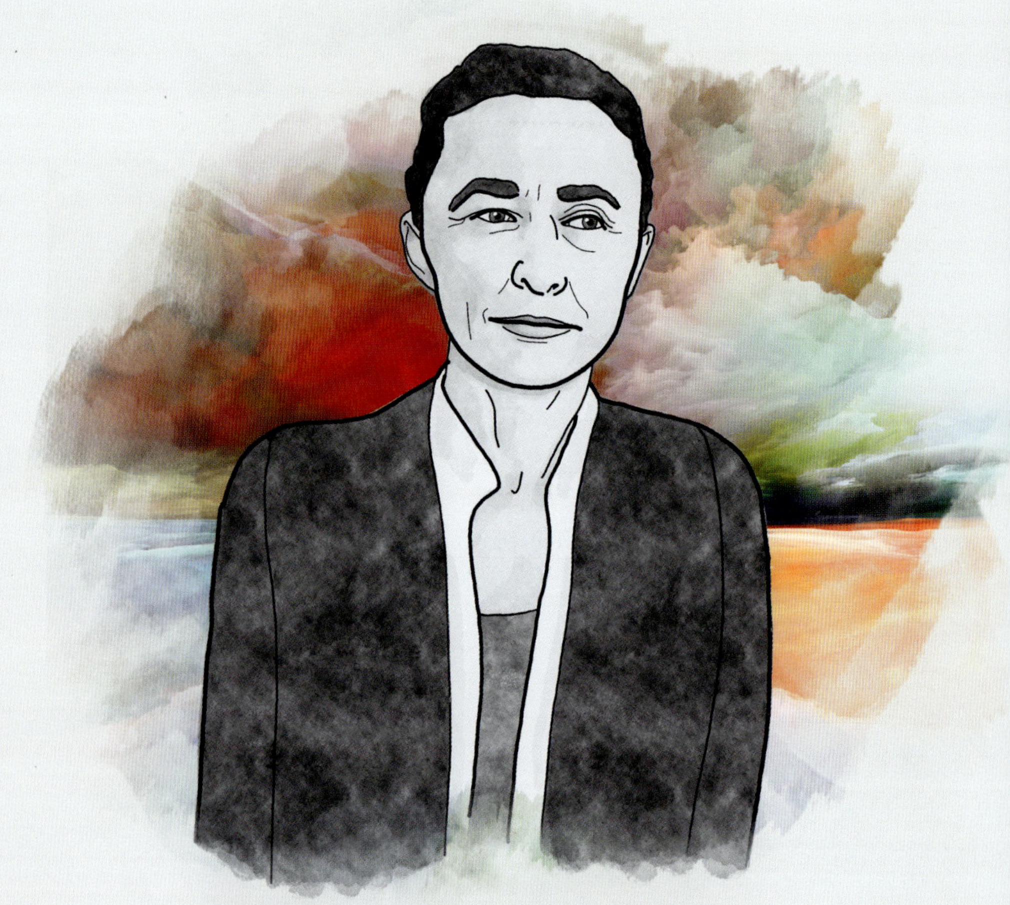

Georgia O'Keeffe

(November 15, 1887–March 6, 1986)

I've always been absolutely terrified every single moment of my life, and I've never let it stop me from doing a single thing I wanted to do.

—GEORGIA O'KEEFFE[1]

Depression is one of the most prevalent mental health issues in the world, second only to anxiety.[2] Georgia O'Keeffe had the unfortunate reality of living with both conditions, which isn't at all uncommon. Also, like many people today, she seemed to have **low-grade (also called "high functioning") forms**, with the exception of one period of major depression that came following a traumatic period of romantic turmoil. O'Keeffe's story is an inspirational one and demonstrates **the importance of radical self-care and thoughtful life choices in order to live peacefully with mental health issues**. By prioritizing herself and her art over a controlling, philandering husband and taxing work environment in New York City, O'Keeffe was able to slow down, breathe deeply, and truly appreciate the beauty of nature. Through her creative meditations on her southwestern desert home, O'Keeffe found an inner quietude that mirrored the desert's tranquility, and she shared it with the world through her paintings.

As a young artist, Georgia O'Keeffe struggled with her sense of self and used her artwork as a form of investigative self-expression. As Sharyn R. Udall phrases it, O'Keeffe made "lifelong efforts . . . to define an artistic style while living out her own invented, unique, and sometimes conflicted personal mythology."[3] In addition to experiencing depression and anxiety, O'Keeffe suffered physical ailments that, as with other artists we've discussed, exacerbated her emotional challenges. These illnesses included typhoid at eighteen, which caused "low spirits," and both rheumatism and breast cancer in 1928. O'Keeffe was also engaged in a turbulent decades-long relationship with high-profile photographer Alfred Stieglitz, who in many ways inspired her art career but who also contributed to her emotional ups and downs.[4]

The romance between Stieglitz and O'Keeffe began as an affair when he was fifty-three and she was thirty. The two were discovered by Stieglitz's wife, Emmy, during a risqué photo session, an event that effectively ended Stieglitz's marriage and estranged him from his adult daughter, Kitty, who would go on to be institutionalized for severe depression and schizophrenia. His family blamed the affair for Kitty's condition, and O'Keeffe bore the burden of Stieglitz's guilt, his emotions overshadowing her own desires during important life decisions. O'Keeffe did not want to marry but begrudgingly acquiesced to wed Stieglitz when doctors thought their union might help Kitty process the dissolution of her own parents' marriage. And though she wanted to become a mother, Stieglitz refused, afraid that history would repeat itself and his actions would harm another child. He perhaps wasn't altogether misguided in this prediction, since years later he would abandon O'Keeffe for a much-younger woman, photographer Dorothy Norman. Stieglitz's affair obviously wasn't easy for O'Keeffe. She went to stay with her sister, where she suffered a racing heart, ongoing headaches, and crying jags, all symptoms of both anxiety and depression. By early 1933, O'Keeffe had checked herself into a hospital for treatment. She was diagnosed with "psychoneurosis," meaning she had emotions pent up that lacked the necessary expressive outlets, which had manifested into physical symptoms.[5] O'Keeffe stopped painting for about a year as she struggled through this time. This is what depression can do: take away an artist's ability to create. **Art can be a source of catharsis, self-esteem, and strength, but depression can overtake and immobilize an artist to the point where they cannot work on their craft**. This may result in feelings of hopelessness and worthlessness, all coalescing into a major creative block.

The upside to this difficult time of her life was that O'Keeffe connected with several other women artists who were going through similar psychological and romantic challenges. She corresponded with Frida Kahlo, who had recently been hospitalized after her miscarriage.[6] The two stayed friends for decades, and O'Keeffe visited Kahlo twice in her Mexico home. O'Keeffe also traveled with photographer Marjorie

Content, who was in the midst of ending her own marriage.[7] One of the most important factors in overcoming depression is a strong support system, and it's likely that O'Keeffe's connections to these women helped immensely in her healing process. O'Keeffe also offered this kind of emotional support to others. When a young Yayoi Kusama sent a letter to O'Keeffe seeking mentorship, O'Keeffe responded with kindness and generous advice for the artist. As we'll see in the chapter about Kusama, the two connected over their shared anxiety.

Even though anxiety is the most prevalent mental health condition in the world, depression is the leading cause of disability. Depression, once romanticized in the arts as a form of "heroic melancholy," in reality frequently erodes the ability to create. Whereas depression saps your ability to create, anxiety can, at times, facilitate art making. Of course, this depends greatly on the individual. For example, anxiety is often characterized by insomnia and restlessness, and many artists find it helpful to channel that sleepless energy into their work. That said, sometimes anxiety manifests as distressing physical symptoms (sweating, shaking, nausea, headaches, muscle pain) and can, along with the symptom of insomnia, lead to extreme feelings of tiredness, which of course renders art making hard.

High-functioning anxiety is not a recognized medical diagnosis but is commonly accepted as a form of anxiety in which the person is often highly successful, though that success is fueled by the anxiety itself. The person is high achieving, detail oriented, outgoing, and otherwise the outward picture of "put together," but they're like a duck paddling furiously in the pond—underneath the calm water their thoughts and emotions are going at a painfully rapid pace. One common feature of high-functioning anxiety is perfectionism, which can lead to procrastination resulting from a fear that the work won't be good enough. This results in a cycle of not working, being forced into an intense "crunch time," followed by a period of burnout.[8] O'Keeffe seems to have been a victim of this cycle. Udall writes, "O'Keeffe's later bouts of depression were often linked to intense work, followed by predictable exhaustion and illness." In a 1917 letter, O'Keeffe writes of this emotional turbulence: "Everything seems to be whirling or unbalanced—I'm suspended in the air—can't get my feet off the ground."[9]

One of the ways that O'Keeffe seems to have self-regulated her anxiety was by spending time in quiet, rural areas. For a six-year period starting in 1912, she took teaching positions in Texas and South Carolina.

Later, of course, her name would become practically synonymous with New Mexico. Although she would spend significant portions of time in New York throughout her life, O'Keeffe would escape to the Southwest for three to six months of each year. As journalist Olivia Laing puts it, "She chafed against the landscape, the noise, the requirements of sociability."[10] The frenetic pace of urban living can exacerbate anxiety for many people. O'Keeffe may have intuitively known that in order to limit anxiety's role in her life, she needed to reduce the triggers of the city and find a place where she could rest both her body and mind.

Using rural retreats as intermittent periods of respite sometimes failed O'Keeffe as a solution to her worries, though. People with anxiety tend to avoid the things that trigger them, which may only serve to intensify their symptoms when they must eventually face their fears. O'Keeffe's coping mechanism of temporary vacations from her life didn't always work. In the 1920s, O'Keeffe's troubles seemed to be directly related to her unstable relationship with Stieglitz. He accompanied her one summer to Lake George, New York, a place that usually brought her peace of mind. This year, however, she described herself as "anxiety-ridden," reporting that she had "lost 15 pounds and was terribly nervous."[11] Despite his pleas, she left him there for a month and went to another rural retreat in Maine, this time alone. This repeated in 1928, when again, after just two weeks at Lake George with Stieglitz, she fled to Maine to be alone. The following year, she wrote in a letter to a friend, "If I can keep my courage and leave Steiglitz I plan to go West."[12] During this turbulent time, she wasn't satisfied with any of the art that she created. She had a 1929 show exhibiting a series of leaf studies with "torn, broken, or jagged edges," which Udall compares to O'Keeffe's feelings, which were "battered and bruised as well."[13] Her short reprieves from the city were no longer sufficient distractions from the unhappiness she felt in her marriage and the stress over her career. Disappointed in herself (recall that being overly self-critical is a trait of high-functioning anxiety), O'Keeffe finally hit a breaking point. That year was the first she spent an extended stay in New Mexico. Away from the East Coast and independent from her husband, O'Keeffe regained a sense of herself. She returned from this trip feeling strong and, in her words, "so alive that I am apt to crack at any moment."[14]

A few short years later, in 1932, O'Keeffe accepted a mural commission for Radio City Hall in New York City. Perhaps due to her anxious perfectionism, she procrastinated the work. With only six weeks left to complete the mural, she arrived to find the wall space hadn't been properly prepared. Overwhelmed, she backed out of the project, a decision she felt guilty and stressed about.[15] As Laing notes, "She couldn't eat and wept for days on end. New York's crowded streets were suddenly appalling, and she became agoraphobic."[16]

By year's end, O'Keeffe was severely anxious and depressed. She was placed on bed rest and improved but then attempted another exhibition in early 1933, which spiked her anxiety right at the time that Stieglitz's affair with Dorothy Norman was also reaching its peak. The culmination of these stressors led to a nervous breakdown, after which O'Keeffe spent two months in a psychiatric hospital. Afterward, she further recuperated in Bermuda, and then at Lake George, where she described feeling a "suffering in my nerves."[17]

O'Keeffe emerged from this experience triumphantly, finally able to work again by 1934 and practicing extreme self-care in regard to protecting her time and energy. She developed a stronger sense of self that motivated her to take control of her own career and stop relying on Stieglitz. Of course, she was not infallible, and recovery is often nonlinear and at times imperfect. But she continued to prioritize her own happiness. She gained financial independence from Stieglitz, and though they remained legally married until his death, O'Keeffe spent an increasing amount of time in New Mexico (until eventually moving there permanently), gaining emotional independence from her husband as well.

Learning to slow down and intentionally minimize chaos in her life helped O'Keeffe manage her depression and anxiety. Giving advice to a friend, O'Keeffe writes: "You wear out the most precious things you have by letting your emotions and feelings run riot . . . we need to conserve our energies." Maintaining this sense of calm was also critical to her success as a painter. Author Maria Popova describes the unusual, up-close perspective of the subjects of her famous flower paintings as "a way of removing the blinders with which we gallop through the world, slowing down, shedding our notions and concepts of things, and taking things in as they really are."[18] Living a simpler life in New Mexico quieted O'Keeffe's negative and racing thoughts and allowed her to hone a unique artistic vision. To quote Olivia Laing, the desert was "nourishing, but part of its nourishment was the way everything was pared back to essentials, the flab cut away."

O'Keeffe's last great series of work came in the 1960s, when, despite a decades-long fascination with stuff of the earth (desert sand, flowers, bones), O'Keeffe took to painting the sky. The works in the *Sky Above Clouds* series are enormous, much bigger than any of her previous paintings, with the largest measuring 24 feet long.[19] It's almost as if O'Keeffe pared down her artistic focus more and more, until all that was left to express were these meditations on the peaceful and expansive nothingness above—a vast blue space, with plenty of room to breathe.

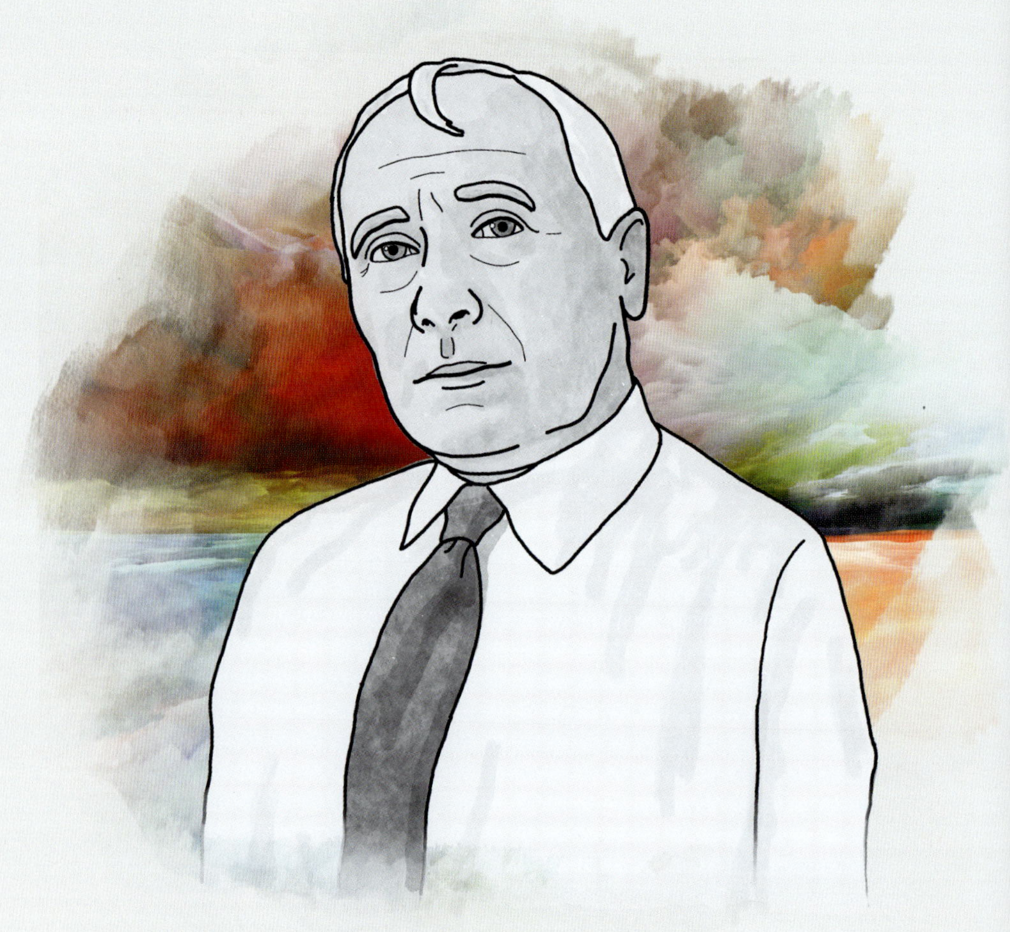

Joan Miró

(April 20, 1893–December 25, 1983)

If we do not attempt to discover the magic sense of things, we will do no more than add new sources of degradations to those already offered to people today, which are beyond number.

—JOAN MIRÓ

Not only did Joan Miró share the fact he suffered from depression widely through his own letters and interviews, but subsequent biographers and critics have done detailed analyses of the role his depression played in relation to his artistic output. This gives us a wealth of information to draw from regarding Miró's personal experience with the condition, as well as a more universal understanding of how art can play a healing role in the life of someone with chronic, recurring depression. In fact, the artist is so well recognized in the field of art and mental health that in the early 1990s, during the centenary celebration exhibit of Miró's work at his foundation in Barcelona, the Catalan Society of Psychiatry held an interdisciplinary symposium on "Mood Disorders and Spirituality in 20th-Century Artists."[1]

Miró's earliest known bout of depression occurred at the age of eighteen, and he basically stayed in bed for an entire season of that year.[2] Even before that major depressive period, Miró was a melancholy youth. He has said that he felt lonely and isolated throughout his childhood and frequently described himself as a pessimist, as though depression were his inevitable state of being. As biographer and friend Roland Penrose describes it: "Behind the cheerful, innocent, even tranquil look in his face, Miró has never been immune to attacks of violent anguish and depression."[3] Miró recalls that he used drawing to cope with that first depressive episode when he was a teen.[4] In a 1947 interview, he said that when he doesn't paint, he gets "black ideas" that lead to worry and gloominess, suggesting that when he does paint, these symptoms are eased.[5] Psychiatric researcher Dr. Joseph Schildkraut, who had a lifelong interest in Miró's art and mental health, believed that art "served as an escape for the Spanish artist and healed his soul."[6]

Ironically, Miró's work is often described as whimsical, or even humorous. Stanley Meiser writes in *Smithsonian* magazine, "It is hard to enter a room full of Mirós without breaking into a smile and feeling a dollop of joy."[7] In the 1960s, an exhibition of thirteen Miró paintings alongside thirteen Alexander Calder mobiles was called "the happiest exhibition of the season."[8] How intriguing that his artwork elicits such a cheerful response when the artist himself felt morose so much of the time. In a 1960s interview, transcribed into the book *Joan Miró: I Work Like a Gardener*, the artist explains that any humor that appears in his work is accidental, an unconscious result of "the need I feel to escape the tragic side of my temperament."[9]

However, sometimes the darkness peeks through. In the 1930s, money was tight due to the Great Depression, and Spain was in the throes of its civil war, and the uncertainty of the times greatly affected Miró. It showed in his work, as he tried to paint through the difficulty of "a heaviness in the head, aching bones and asphyxiating dampness."[10] One of his most famous paintings from this time is *Still Life with Old Shoe*, which some have compared to Picasso's *Guernica*, identifying the abandoned shoe (and other details, such as a fork stabbed into an apple) as symbols of the horrors of war. Again skirting the topic of intention, Miró said he didn't consciously paint the war, only that he knew that he was painting something deeply serious. He confesses, though, that he almost couldn't finish the painting because of a "general feeling of terror" that overtook him.[11] Again we see world events impacting both an artist's mental health and their art.

In the year before the creation of *Still Life with Old Shoe*, he painted *Man and Woman in Front of a Pile of Excrement*, in which the anguish of his life experience is expressed through the strangeness of the figures, their garish yellow skin contrasting starkly against the impenetrable blackness of the background. It was painted as Spain was on the precipice of war, and seems to express a violent anxiety. And yet, though not as lighthearted as some of his other works, this painting is not entirely devoid of Miró's particular brand of humor; it has even been called a "dark comedy."[12] Perhaps art critic Michael Gibson got it right when he wrote of Miró, "Humor, as opposed to sarcasm and certain forms of irony, also appears to be rooted in an indestructible region of the artist's humanity. It clears the ground to build something of its own: in this case, a more satisfactory metaphorical world."[13] Miró himself explained his choice of title: "I was obsessed by Rembrandt's words: 'I find rubies and emeralds in a dung heap,'" suggesting **the power of art making to find meaning in life's many misfortunes.**[14]

A few years later, during World War II, Miró and his wife went into hiding in her hometown of Majorca. With the world collapsing around him, the artist wondered if he would ever work as a painter again. Yet, during this dark time, he painted *The Constellations*, a unique series of work that he smuggled out of Europe to exhibit in the United States. Exhibited stateside in 1945, it was one of America's first signs that European art was still thriving—a beacon of hope.[15] Struggling to cope with the tragedy of a world at war, he was able to transmute his personal depression into art that connected cultures—finding rubies, so to speak.[16]

Although Miró was open about coping with depression, his family felt the stigma of the condition. When psychiatrist Dr. Joseph Schildkraut published a book analyzing Miró's art through the lens of depression, his family members "weren't too happy," though Miró's grandson did contact the doctor to confirm the diagnosis.[17] Additionally, some find Schildkraut's interpretations of depression disorders in artists controversial. He argued that depression turns you inward and, in many ways, makes an artistic calling "easier." The doctor even goes so far as to say that depression in artists is beneficial to the larger public because of the great art it engenders.[18] But what about all of the artists who simply cannot create during depressive periods, or those lost to depressive disorders due to substance abuse issues or suicide? There are many different aspects to consider when we look at the intersection of art and mental health. **Do Miró's artistic contributions to the world offset the cost of his suffering?** It's not an easy question to answer.

In a 1965 interview with Yvon Taillandier, Miró states, "When a painting doesn't satisfy me, I feel physical distress, as if ill, as if my heart isn't working properly, as if I can't breathe and am suffocating." He goes on to say that the entire process is a struggle, a battle between himself and his anxieties that he works out on the canvas: "This struggle is passionately exciting to me. I work until the distress leaves me."[19] So, while an unsatisfactory piece may cause him distress, achieving his creative vision soothes his mind. When a piece is completed to his satisfaction, at least for that moment, the worries evaporate. He has painted them away. Miró considered his paintings a garden, and himself their gardener. He tended to his canvases like plants, beginning with the germination of ideas, putting down roots, and allowing them to grow. He didn't mind having canvases in progress for years, sometimes working on them sporadically and other times simply letting them sit. After all, it takes time to reap what you have sown. Given his previous statement about distress, one might suspect that having unfinished work would be an issue for the artist. However, if he felt that he was at a good stopping point, and that the natural next step was to rest for a time, he was happy to have "growing" things around him in his studio.[20]

This practice may also shed some light upon Miró's experience of depression. The artist seemed to have cycles of productivity, experiencing very rich periods of constant work, followed by depressive episodes during which he couldn't paint at all and had many subtle ups and downs in between. One argument made about Miró is that although he was never diagnosed as having bipolar depression, he might have had **cyclothymia.**[21] On the depression spectrum, this sits somewhere in the middle—the individual has periods of depression, but usually not major depressive episodes, and also has periods of hypomania, though never rising to the full heights of bipolar mania. Miró himself wrote about the phases of his life and work, describing consistent, recurring cycles that affected both his rate of productivity and the painting process itself.[22] When we consider the garden metaphor for his studio in this light, we can see that perhaps his ups and downs—working through the distress of beginning a painting, getting it to an acceptable state, and letting it sit for a time before picking it up again—are indicative of more than just the creative process; it's possible this pattern is directly linked with his cyclothymic depression rhythms.

Miró found a way to live with his depressive cycles for well over eight decades, and art may well have been what helped him cope. It also seems that his depressive states, and other life experiences, may have given Miró an empathy and appreciation for humanity that he was able to express through painting. He has said that "the thing I consciously seek is tension in spirit," alluding to the interplay of his mental health struggles and creative drive.[23] The way in which Miró channeled his fear, exasperation, and sadness to produce joyful and charismatic paintings, to which so many people relate, shows us that **art has the power not only to help the individual artist cope with depression, but also to connect us all to our shared humanity.**

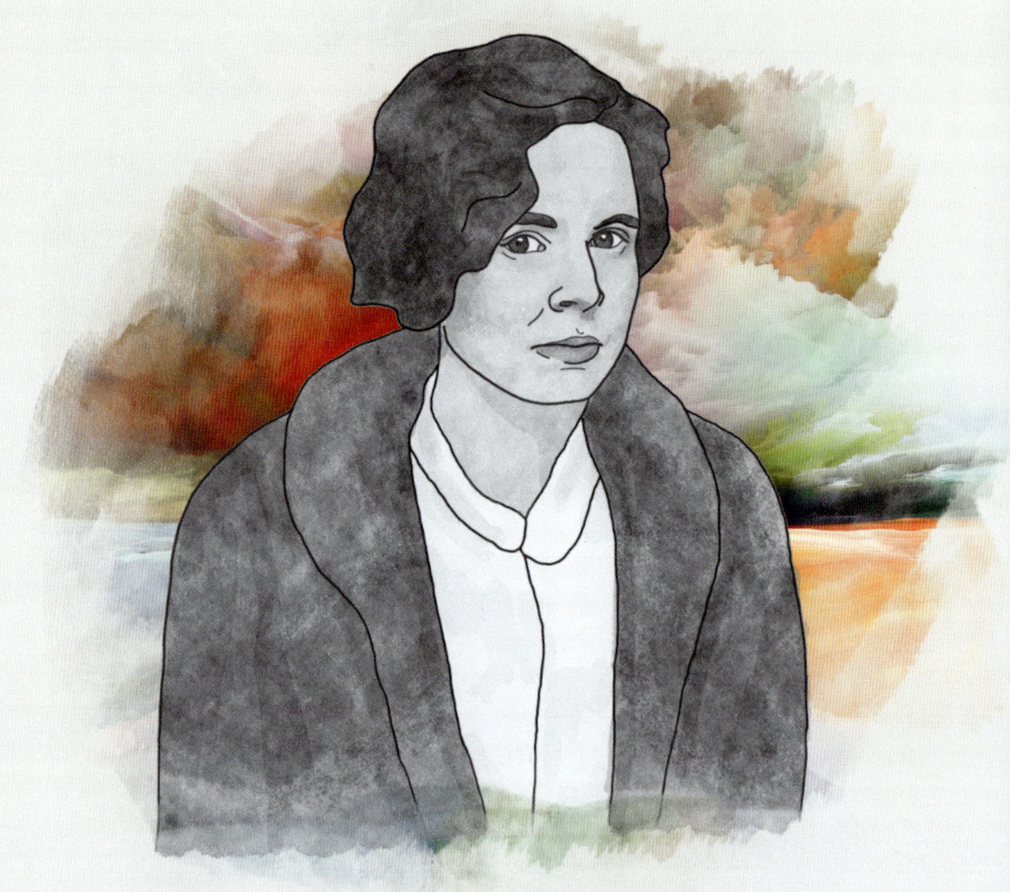

Alice Neel

(January 28, 1900–October 13, 1984)

If I don't paint for certain lengths of time, I get into frightfully morbid moods, but the minute I begin to work, I'm cured. Sometimes though, after I've finished a painting, I feel like an untenanted house, utterly alone.

–ALICE NEEL[1]

As we will address in the next section, trauma often plays a role in mental health issues. Childhood trauma, the trauma of war, or any number of other significant events can be deeply intertwined with mental health symptoms. In some cases, a person is diagnosed from the trauma itself, posttraumatic stress disorder (PTSD) being the classic example. However, **depression can also be related to underlying trauma.** This may have been the case for Alice Neel, an artist who struggled with major depression (also called **unipolar depression**) yet became famous for her intimate, empathic portraits of friends and family, and honest artistic portrayals of her life's struggles.

Before the age of thirty, Neel lost a child to diphtheria and was abandoned by her husband, the influential Cuban artist Carlos Enríquez. Their daughter, Santillana, died of the disease before her first birthday in 1927. The following year, shortly after the birth of their second daughter, Isabetta, Enríquez left for Cuba, taking the child with him. Neel was under the assumption that the situation was temporary, and that she would meet her husband in Paris while Isabetta stayed with her aunts in Cuba, and didn't expect to be separated from her daughter for long. However, Neel would not see her daughter for six years.[2] The experience of losing her first child was devastating, and losing another child to separation nearly broke her. Although she initially threw herself into painting in an attempt to work through the sadness, Neel ultimately had a breakdown and was hospitalized.[3] Released from the hospital after a few months, she attempted suicide by sticking her head in the oven shortly after.[4] She was rehospitalized and made a second suicide attempt by attempting to swallow shards of glass, but luckily her attendants were able to intervene.[5]

When looking to Neel's art as a reflection of her state of mind, it seems possible she was suffering even before the events of that summer. *Well Baby Clinic*, which she painted two weeks after the birth of her second daughter, depicts a baby in the arms of a nurse, the duo surrounded by bleak characters. A painting of a newborn's birth would presumably be joyful, and yet, this work—with mostly unattended-to infants surrounding the child in the center—seems to foreshadow the mood of paintings she would later make of her time in the asylum. Another work, *Requiem*, painted in memory of her daughter who died, is a dark depiction of skeletal creatures in a storm that has often been compared with Edvard Munch's *The Scream*.

Neel had been an artist for as long as she could remember and had mental health challenges since she was a child. She was diagnosed at a young age with **neurasthenia**, the vague term popular at the time to describe a set of symptoms we now recognize as signs of depression. It was generally women who were diagnosed with neurasthenia, and extreme bed rest was the suggested cure. But for Neel, art was the cure. Although she didn't take art classes in school, she always loved drawing, coloring, and painting and knew from experience that creating helped her mood.

Neel very much wanted to paint while she was in the asylum but was forbidden from painting while first hospitalized.[6] Art has played a changing role in therapy over the course of history, at times celebrated and utilized as a tool but at other times devalued and disallowed. Luckily for Alice Neel, and for the world, a social worker eventually took an interest in her, learned about her love of art, and offered her a drawing pad—a gesture that may have saved her life.

Often, Neel created biographical art as a means of processing the trauma she was currently experiencing. It has frequently been noted that her life and work are seemingly inseparable. Writer Grace Glueck calls Neel's life "a saga whose chapters she committed to paint almost as fast as they unfolded."[7] Take a look at *Futility of Effort*, which she painted in 1930. A lifeless body hangs off the bed in a gray room that is sparse and empty. It's a direct representation of the loss of her child, and the hopelessness she felt as she dealt with that grief. *Degenerate Madonna*, also painted in 1930, is of a ghostly and unhappy-looking woman holding an eerie-looking child, while another's silhouette lingers in the background. If art is a means of processing grief and loss, this seems to be a direct attempt to move through the pain of losing her children. Despite being an intensely personal piece, *Degenerate Madonna* elicited such outrage from the Catholic Church due to its title that she had to withdraw it from the first Washington Square Outdoor Art Exhibit.[8]

Similarly biographical, *Suicidal Ward* (1931) is a visual expression of what it was like for Neel to be hospitalized. Asylums and other institutions for mental health vary widely in terms of the kind of care they give, informed by a variety of factors including the scientific and sociocultural beliefs of the times, the funding afforded the institutions, and the amount of oversight they receive. Phoebe Hoban's 2010 book about Neel describes the asylum as "horrifying," from the painful spinal epidural Neel was given upon arrival, to the monotony of 5 a.m. breakfasts with rubber utensils, not to mention the toll of living among patients in varied states of distress. Neel reportedly longed for oblivion and contemplated suicide daily, and *Suicidal Ward* is a visual depiction of this despair.

Nevertheless, Neel found her refuge in art making. "It was drawing that helped me decide to get well," she said.[9] Eventually, she was able to move from the Philadelphia General Hospital to a private sanitarium, the Gladwyne Colony, where she received better treatment and began the long process of recovery.[10] Gladwyne, created by innovative psychiatrist Dr. Seymour DeWitt Ludlum, used a wide variety of therapeutic treatments, from craft (or occupational) therapy to electroshock. Neel found the place healing, creating for herself a therapeutic ritual of taking long baths, reading books, and making art. Imagine if she had been stuck with that earlier diagnosis of neurasthenia and forced instead to stay in bed motionless for a month. She might never have survived. In addition to crediting her art with saving her, she also credits her therapist, Dr. Anthony Sterrett, who she began psychotherapy with in 1958, decades after she left the asylum. And, bravely, Neel also credits herself. Author Joan Kufrin shares that Neel told her that, ultimately, you are the one that has to decide to try to get well. You will need help to do it, but you must make the decision and do the work.[11]

Neel did the work and eventually got healthier and was able to leave the hospital. Shortly thereafter, she fell in love with José Santiago

Negrón, with whom she had a son. Then, Negrón left her for a younger woman, triggering her issues of abandonment from her first husband and the loss of her two daughters. Neel put all of her feelings into her artwork, and her portraits of José from the 1930s have been called sullen, pensive, and brooding. As writer Helen Harrison puts it, "The anxiety, distress and anomie of her subjects mirrored the problems of her private life."[12] Harrison goes on to note that although Neel is best known for her portraits, a look at the settings of the paintings—empty streets, empty rooms, and hospital wards—gives deeper insight into the artist's depression. One of the most powerful works of art from this time is a symbolic still life of Negrón's guitar hanging over a potted plant. Her sadness is palpable, and the title of the piece, *Loneliness*, is reinforced by the fact that no humans appear in the picture—only a memory of him remains.

Alice Neel was well known for her nude portraits and particularly enjoyed painting nudes of pregnant women. She revisited the subject repeatedly but never let the universal experience eclipse the individual one. "While one might seem burdened by her belly, as in *Pregnant Betty Homitzky* (1968), another looks frankly sensual, as in *Pregnant Julie and Algis* (1964), in which a naked woman lies beside her clothed partner on a rumpled bedspread."[13] Perhaps ruminating on the experience of pregnancy offered continued catharsis for Neel, who experienced miscarriages as well as the death of her first daughter.[14] Or, perhaps it was a reflection of her deep understanding of the strength it took to choose to be a mother, especially a single mother, during a time when women's roles were drastically changing. Neel was certainly aware of the great progress made in the women's liberation movement. She was in her teens and twenties during women's suffrage and well into her sixties when the women's revolution came about, so a lot of ground was covered in her lifetime. Neel was even asked to paint the portrait of famous feminist Kate Millet for the 1970 cover of *TIME* magazine.[15] Living her life as an independent single mother who supported herself through her art was revolutionary in and of itself.

Although society often deems depression as a personal problem, looking through a broader lens often reveals an intersection between societal issues and individual mental health problems. Alice Neel's own depression was intricately tied up with her social conscience. In 1933, she painted *Investigation of Poverty at the Russell Sage Foundation* and *Synthesis of New York—the Great Depression*, both of which clearly reflect the widespread economic devastation of the times.[16] A few years later, she painted *Nazis Murder Jews*, an unequivocally political painting that reflects the trauma of the era.[17] Like Joan Miró's *Man and Woman in Front of a Pile of Excrement*, it's an artistic response that gives us insight on how it might have felt to live during those events. Twenty years later, she painted *Eisenhower, McCarthy, Dulles*, a harsh commentary on Cold War politics.[18] Just as we cannot separate Neel's art from her life, neither can we separate her personal symptoms of depression from the upheaval occurring in the world around her.

Neel went on to live into her eighties without another suicide attempt. However, in her older years, she described herself as having been suicidal for most of her life. It is critical to understand this component of depression. Some people experience a period of depression that lasts for a brief time and then never returns. However, many people experience persistent depressive disorder, also called **dysthymia**, which is depression that lasts for two years or more at a time. That's two years when most days of the week you feel hopeless and worthless, lack energy, and might not wish to live at all. We can't begin to imagine the struggles Neel endured—surviving years of depression, hospitalization, suicide attempts, abusive relationships, and the death of a child. We can, however, marvel at the power and potential of art making, each of her paintings a reminder to persevere through challenging times.

Artists and Suicide

The link between creativity and mood disorders is not exactly clear from a scientific perspective for many reasons. One is the difficulty of defining "creativity" in a way that is measurable from a statistical standpoint. Another difficulty lies in identifying an appropriate control group; since mental illness[1] can be influenced by so many factors, it's not easy to isolate creativity when studying the relationship between the two. However, the sheer number of studies undertaken on the subject shows that researchers have reason to believe there is a correlation between creativity and mood disorders, and depression and suicide specifically.

One theory for why suicide may be more prevalent in these groups is that making art can be an antisocial and isolating practice, a "dangerous surrogate and addiction" that takes the place of healthy habits and caring for one's mental health.[2] Often, due to lack of enrichment in other areas of their lives, artists base too much of their self-worth on their creative output. Should their depression worsen or some other factor impede their ability to make art, life may not seem worth living.

In contradiction, art therapy has grown in popularity as a method to help people who are at risk of dying by suicide. So, what's the difference? Studies suggest that making art can be useful in this context, but not necessarily if it is self-guided. Art therapy has proven most effective when it is included as part of a class or program specifically designed to diminish suicide risk or alleviate depression. This means that the artmaking could be accompanied by group discussion, mental health education, and even individual cognitive therapy.[3] The differentiating factor seems to be, simply, other people. Social interaction is vital to people experiencing suicidal ideation—how often do we hear of someone who died by suicide having felt lonely or misunderstood? Furthermore, art can be a valuable tool allowing people to express thoughts or emotions for which they cannot find words, whether that be because of social stigma or people simply not having the tools to verbalize their feelings.

A creative outlet can truly be a lifesaver for someone suffering with depression, so long as they are not weathering the storm alone.

If you or someone you know needs help, the 988 Suicide & Crisis Lifeline is available 24/7. Simply call or text 988 or visit 988lifeline.org/chat

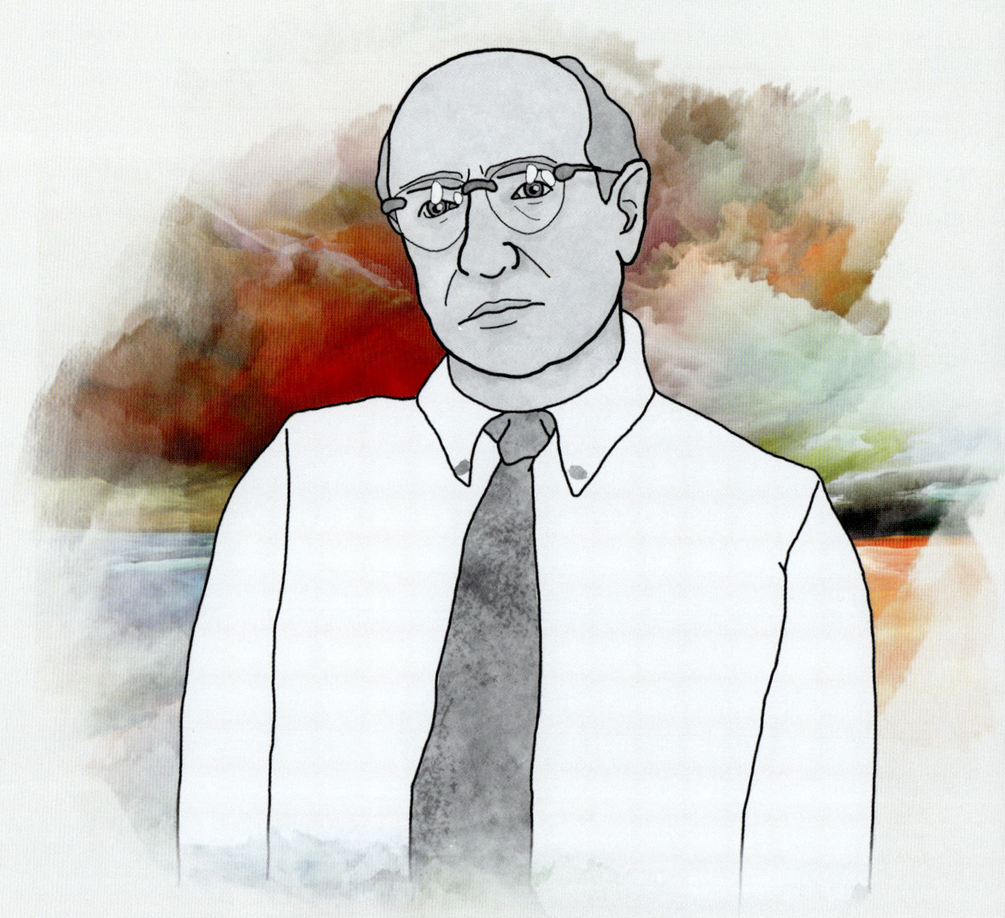

Mark Rothko

(September 25, 1903–February 25, 1970)

To us art is an adventure into an unknown world, which can be explored only by those willing to take the risk.

—MARK ROTHKO[1]

Mark Rothko is known for his monumental abstract paintings consisting of vast fields of colors that, in their simplicity, evoke the sublime experience of living—the sadness and tragedy, as well as the meaningful universal connections. In this chapter we will explore how early childhood loss, intergenerational trauma, and spirituality stemming from his Jewish faith all coalesced into Rothko's art. We will also see how his depression disorder hindered the artist creatively and rendered happiness elusive, with the culmination of Rothko's life tragically from suicide.

Rothko didn't have the easiest start in life. He was the youngest child of aging parents, born (as Marcus Rothkovich) into a Jewish ghetto in Russia under a czarist government.[2] Just one example of the devastation from this era was on June 1, 1906, when two hundred Jewish people died and another seven hundred were injured in a pogrom meant to massacre Russian Jews. When Mark was an infant, his father, who had previously not been particularly religious, felt compelled to refocus on his Jewish faith in response to the death surrounding him. Whereas Mark's siblings attended secular schools, Mark began studying at a Talmudic school at the age of four. When Rothko was seven, his father left for America in search of a better life for his family. He sent for Mark's older brothers soon after, but Mark and his mother didn't join them until three years later, in 1913.[3] When they finally reunited in the US, Mark struggled with the transition. Tragically, his father died of colon cancer just months after their arrival.[4]

The Rothkos lived in Portland, Oregon, where they had extended family and strong community ties, but Mark always felt out of place. The young Rothko struggled to learn the language and to fit in with his peers. In adulthood he would say, "I was never able to forgive this transplantation to a land where I never felt entirely at home."[5] Creative from a young age, as he grew older Rothko also felt that Portland was lacking an artistic community. A diligent student, he went to Yale, but he was stigmatized socially there for being Jewish and he ultimately dropped out.[6] Although Rothko would go on to become well recognized among a circle of New York artists as an adult, his children would later say that he never stopped feeling like an outcast.[7]

Friends frequently described Rothko as melancholy or despondent, even when things were going well in his life.[8] And unfortunately, oftentimes things were not going well at all. Rothko started teaching art in 1929, a job he never liked but continued to do for three decades—even after becoming a recognized artist—because it provided a steady, consistent paycheck. In the early years, his decision to teach was due in large part to pressure from his wife, Edith, who was practical minded and didn't particularly support his art career.[9] She insisted that in addition to teaching, he take on various menial odd jobs, which he abhorred, and she criticized him for his attention to art in ways that he found both frustrating and demeaning.[10] They divorced in the early 1940s; interestingly, despite her rejection of his career as an artist, she accepted a number of his paintings as part of the divorce settlement.

Although their relationship had its faults, the end of the marriage was hard on Rothko.[11] Even before the divorce, there was at least one period of separation initiated by Edith. When she left, Rothko took to his bed in a state of deep depression, speaking endlessly about how humiliated and upset he was by the ordeal.[12] **A ruminating mind is a hallmark of depression**—the brain repeats the same thoughts over and over with no resolution, getting more upset with time. Rothko's brain latched on to the shame he felt over being left by his wife, and had trouble letting go.

When they divorced a few years later, he compared the pain of the divorce to "pulling the skin from his cheek" and checked himself into a hospital for three weeks with a self-induced cancer scare that appears to have been a physical manifestation of his depression.[13] Many people, particularly men, experience depression physically before, or in addition to, recognizing its psychological toll. Backaches, stomach distress, and headaches are the most-common complaints. It's totally within the realm of possibility that these, and other vague symptoms, could snowball into fear of a serious disease, especially if one was already prone to hypochondriacal thoughts. During this depressive period, Rothko couldn't paint.

In 1944, Rothko met the love of his life, Mary Alice (usually called Mell), and they married shortly thereafter. Things were looking up, and his art career started to gain momentum. The same year he and Mary Alice were married, Rothko had a solo show at Peggy Guggenheim's Art of This Century gallery. The following year, Rothko began showing at the Betty Parsons Gallery, and within five years of that he exhibited work at the Museum of Modern Art.[14] In 1958, he represented the United States at the 29th Venice Biennale.[15] He was gaining international recognition, but Rothko still struggled with insecurities, frustration, and depressive periods.

In 1948, Rothko fell into a clinical depression and withdrew from a teaching position as a result.[16] This was due in part to grief over the death of his mother that year.[17] A mother's death is always difficult, but psychiatrists have speculated that the loss was especially hard for Rothko because it echoed the loss of his father—first to immigration and then when he passed away.[18] Rothko wrote of this time that although his paintings might have looked cheery to viewers, he was going through the darkest winter of his life.[19] This harkens back to interpretations of Miró's work as humorous, while the artist himself described it as an unconscious attempt to escape the misery of his own depression.

Rothko's depression, like that of most of our subjects, significantly affected his creative output. It was only when he was feeling relatively emotionally stable that he could find the inspiration to paint. Many artists have their mental health tied up with their creative output, not only in terms of using art as a form of self-expression, but also in linking their sense of self-worth to how well their work is received. Rothko was a progressive artist who caused polarization among critics. He was a critical figure in the abstract expressionist movement, which aimed to create nonrepresentational works that were imbued with emotion, or somehow spoke to the universal human condition. While many were drawn to the new style of painting, others hated it. The *New York Times* wrote about Rothko and his peers: "The pictures are mostly such as to give any one with the slightest academic sympathies apoplexy . . . there is much needless obscurity and reasonless distortion in most of the work."[20]

The human brain tends to dwell on the negative over the positive, and depression makes this pattern of thought even more prevalent. So, even though there were many who praised Rothko for his innovations in painting, he hyperfocused on the criticism. Rothko was obsessed over how rejected he felt by the art world. Interestingly, one of the critiques of his artwork at the time was that it felt empty, which many say was the intent of his calm, contemplative canvases, but which is also a word associated with depression. In reality, since abstract art was so new, many people simply didn't understand what his paintings were trying to say. Art critic Robert Melville wrote in 1957:

> It is baffling and mysterious in its simplicity, and I know that many people only find it an insult to their intelligence; but if by some miracle Rothko's attitude to painting were to prevail, we should all be on the way to becoming converts to Zen Buddhism.[21]

Later, when abstract expressionism became better understood, people began to see a depth of feeling in his juxtaposition of color. But that acceptance would take time, and the negative reviews were hard for Rothko to endure.

It wasn't just the critical reception of his art that plagued the artist. Ironically, the success of his work may have also contributed to his depression. Rothko greatly distrusted material success, particularly in terms of how it could have an impact on his art. Having money seemed to actually cause him distress; he preferred to pay in cash for everything and would reportedly fall into depression whenever he had to go to a bank.

Trying to understand the artist's mental health as it relates to his paintings, many people have suggested that the stylistic progression of his work mirrors his decline into depression. Rothko's final series, *Black on Grey*, seems to mark the worst of his illness.[22] However, years after his death, his daughter, Kate, said she no longer saw it so simply. She notes that in retrospectives of his work, it's easy to compare the bright colors of his 1950s paintings with the dark tones of his later years and see it as depression in action. Though for many years she, too, was unable to separate her father's art from his mental health, Kate now considers his later period as a fresh start for her father—a man with a new way of seeing things.[23] This view is echoed by art dealer Arne Glimcher, who says that what viewers of Rothko's 1950s palette call "sunny and bright," Rothko himself said were "inferno colors" (again, a connection to Joan Miró and the intensity of colors in his "wild paintings"). Glimcher posits that the entirety of Rothko's oeuvre, not only the more somber work from his later years, emanates tragedy.[24]

The complexity of emotion inherent in all of Rothko's art is also recognized by his son, Christopher, who says that his father felt that people didn't understand "the more serious emotional push-pull underneath the color combinations" in his paintings. He says his father switched to a darker palette specifically to better communicate this intensity.[25] Glimcher adds that "painting was a positive, exulting experience for him" and that Rothko attempted to capture on the canvas universal emotions rather than simply echo his own moods.[26] More than a decade prior to his death, Rothko is quoted as saying, "The people who weep before my pictures are having the same religious experience I had when I painted them." Curator Alison de Lima Greene says that if the darkness of his late paintings represents melancholy, "it's closer to the melancholia of Albrecht Dürer, which is a contemplative state rather than a nihilistic one."[27] No one denies that Rothko lived with depression or that there was a relationship between that and his art, but the expression of that relationship is not always as simple as reading a bright painting as "happy" and a dark one as "sad."

After decades of struggling with depression, Rothko had an aneurysm, which precipitated his final bout with the disease.[28] He became particularly despondent as he faced his own mortality and stopped producing art altogether. In the six months prior to his death, he seemed plagued by the feeling both that the art world had rejected his work and simultaneously that the art scene was filled with artists who had been inspired by it. This was a complicated duality that was said to have "consumed him."[29] His ruminating mind repeatedly ran through the same negative thoughts, digging the ruts in the brain deeper, worsening his depression. In those last months, Rothko was mentally exhausted from his internal battle with the art world and his own fame.

There were external battles to be dealt with, as well. Rothko was embroiled in a complicated disagreement over his work with the Marlborough Gallery (a legal battle that would plague his children for years to come). The dispute led to an uncomfortable visit from a gallery representative on the day of his death. Rothko had always preferred to choose which of his work to put up for sale, but this time the agent insisted on making the selections.[30] Rothko had historically been very particular about whom he would allow to buy his work. If a potential buyer didn't seem as if they had a deep understanding of his piece, then he wouldn't sell it to them, at any price. He cared deeply about his art and where it ended up, once saying: "A painting lives by companionship, expanding and quickening in the eyes of the sensitive observer. It dies by the same token. It is therefore a risky and unfeeling act to send it out into the world."[31]

However, on that day, he allowed the gallery representative to choose the paintings, and allowed him to take more than ever before. Had he given away too much of himself that day? From another perspective, people who intend to die by suicide sometimes give away their belongings in advance; it can be a warning sign for family members. Perhaps this change, giving away much more of his work than usual to the Marlborough Gallery agent, was in that vein. Even if that's the case, it doesn't mean he had no regrets; he may have felt devastatingly resigned to this lack of control over where his completed work was headed in the world.

In all likelihood, this event was the final straw in a long series of other factors complicating his depression. By this point, his second marriage was troubled, despite a deep and abiding love between them. They ended up separating, which devastated Rothko. Not only did he feel sadness over the separation, but there were also echoed feelings of abandonment from his first divorce. He was hopeless, with a "desolate outlook on life." He began to talk again about his mother at this time, and the impact her death had on him decades previous. The loss of his wife through separation seems to have triggered the memories of other losses in his life, and in a way forced him to relive the trauma. The grief of the past mingled with the depression of the present in a disastrous conflagration that appears to have been simply too much for the artist to bear.[32]

Rothko's mental health problems were also complicated by his medical issues. In the years preceding his aneurysm, his doctors diagnosed him with cirrhosis and emphysema, citing his copious drinking and smoking as the cause.[33] The artist himself was increasingly alarmed by the effect his substance use was having on his mind and body. However, he also reportedly refused to stop, suggesting an addiction over which he had little control.[34] Moreover, he had an increasing number of other physical and mental complaints, from a hernia that he refused surgery for, to mood swings where he quickly went from "morose and docile" to "agitated and resistant."[35]

Though he didn't always follow their advice, Rothko was seeing several doctors toward the end of his life. Unfortunately, these various doctors were not working together and in fact were often at odds. **Medications can be a lifesaver for some people with depression, but they also have a lot of side effects and risks, especially in regard to interactions with other drugs and alcohol**. This was especially true in the late 1960s, when these medications were not as well understood. It seems that the medications Rothko was taking may have played a role in making his depression worse, rather than better, and his different doctors could not agree on a solution. Reportedly, after not seeing one doctor, Dr. Meade, for over a year, Rothko showed up to his office unannounced, "disoriented, disturbed and dazed." Dr. Meade determined that the psychiatric medication Sinequan was the cause, going further to say that Rothko was "way overmedicated" and that with each dose of the drug his depression and irritability would worsen. Rothko also went "doctor shopping," once seeing multiple doctors until he was prescribed the sleeping pills he desired.[36] The problems Rothko was experiencing may not have simply been with the medication itself, but also the fact that the artist would not take them as prescribed, sometimes missing doses and at other times taking pills a handful at a time.[37] These are medications specifically designed to alter brain chemistry, so to take them in ways that are not prescribed is dangerous and can significantly change a person's thought processing.

In 1969, after he first began taking the psychiatric medication, but before his final six months of depressive inactivity, Rothko spoke about the drug's benefits for his creativity.[38] He noted that he was able to paint again. This excited Rothko, who was happy to be working, despite experiencing fluctuations in his mood. He believed the drug assisted him in regaining his creative energy, which may be why he insisted upon continuing the course of treatment despite other ill effects. Unfortunately, as we know, the surge of creativity did not last, and in the last six months of his life Rothko did not paint at all. Another possible reason for this is that his doctors recommended changes that altered his creative process: he was told not to use turpentine, to switch to acrylics, and to do works that were much smaller in size compared to his previous creations. These all were prescriptions made for the benefit of his health—fewer chemicals, less strain on the body, etc. He abided by these rules, but they certainly affected his experience of making art.

Just before his death by suicide, Rothko was moved to try to paint again. His final work, an untitled piece completed in 1970, is bright red. He had been working in that dark-black and gray palette for some time, so this color was a divergence. Many suggest that it was a foreshadowing of his suicide, which was a violently bloody act.[39] He was found in a room-sized pool of his own blood after having cut an artery in his right arm and taking an overdose of his antidepressant.[40] Perhaps the vivacity of this last red painting was indicative of his desire to feel something, anything, rather than to continue experiencing the bleak numbness of depression.

Research today indicates that **intergenerational trauma** has played a particularly significant role in the psychology of many Jewish people, and though he did not actively practice Judaism, Rothko's experience of life, tragedy, and belonging was deeply connected to his Jewish identity. Anyone whose family experienced the pogroms that devastated the Russian Jewish community in Rothko's youth, or the horrors of the Holocaust that occurred within his lifetime, could be psychologically affected through the ripple effects of trauma in the family, despite not directly experiencing them.

In 1947, Rothko expressed a wish that he had lived in the past, when people could more widely relate to monsters, demons, gods, and nature. He felt as though he was trying to speak to a generation that simply couldn't understand, though he held hope that his message would touch their collective unconscious in some way.[41] In one essay he writes, "Those who believe that the world today is less brutal and ungrateful . . . are either unaware of reality or they do not want to see it in art."[42] Perhaps this summarizes the underlying spirit at the heart of his paintings: the tragedy of the human condition.

How were art and depression linked for Mark Rothko? He used art to express, in his words, "tragedy, ecstasy" and "doom." He used art to find meaning. But when he was most depressed, he could not paint. To create, he would first have to emerge from the darkness—a darkness that was eventually inescapable.

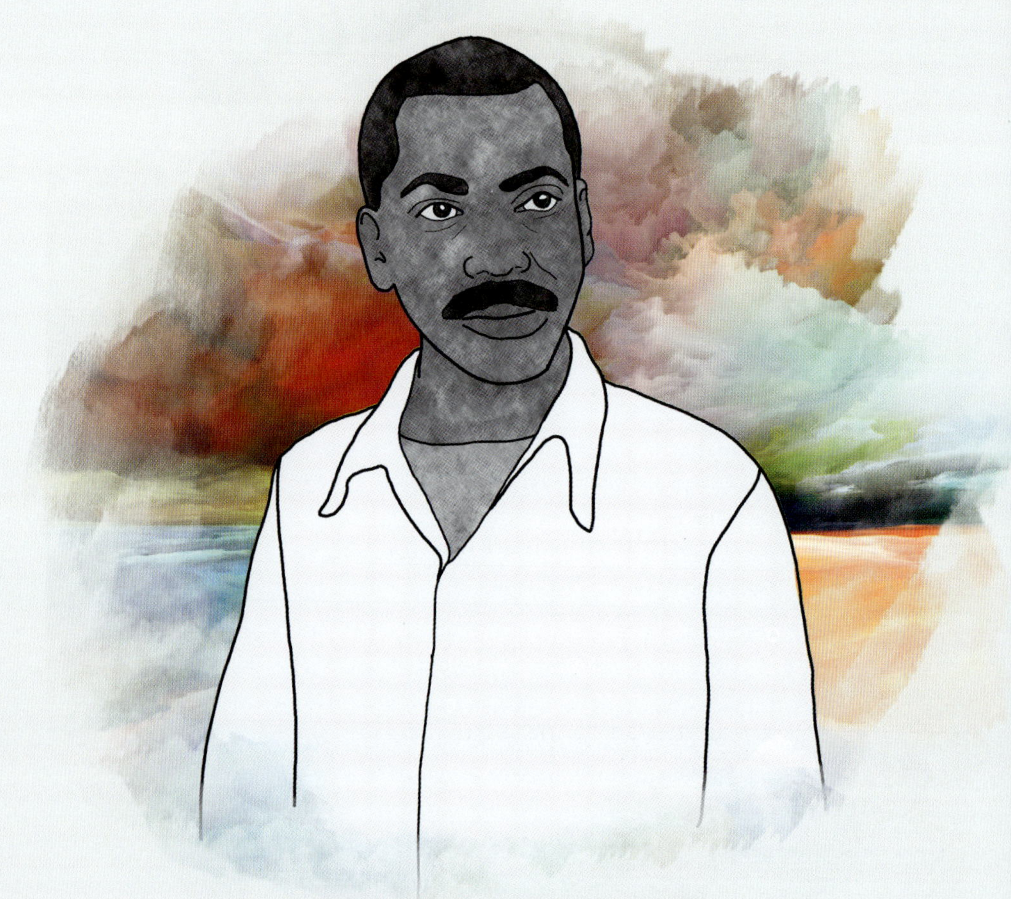

Jacob Lawrence

(September 7, 1917–June 9, 2000)

If at times my productions do not express the conventionally beautiful, there is always an effort to express the universal beauty of man's continuous struggle to lift his social position and to add dimension to his spiritual being.

–JACOB LAWRENCE[1]

Jacob Lawrence is best known for his *Migration* paintings, a sixty-panel series created in his early twenties that depicts struggle but also represents triumph. It is an autobiographical series—the story of his family's move from the South to Harlem—but more than that, the paintings describe the cultural shift of the Great Migration, when African Americans moved to industrialized northern cities starting around 1916. This series, along with much of Lawrence's work, gave narrative and pictorial voice to the stories he found most important, and educated others about issues of race in America.[2]

Lawrence also created art celebrating African American icons, such as Harriet Tubman and Frederick Douglass, and addressed other socially important topics in his art such as war and religion. But there is one specific body of work that stands out from the rest: *The Hospital*, a series of paintings Lawrence created while admitted for inpatient treatment for depression.

The Hospital features scenes from his experience in the asylum and differs not just in subject matter but also in color. The patients are painted in dull and sickly hues and are generally depicted without expression or emotion. It's also notable that most of the figures are white. In the totality of Lawrence's body of work, most of his subjects are Black, so this is a clear departure. Lawrence was struggling with some important questions about race when he fell into the depression that caused him to check himself into a Queens psychiatric hospital.[3] He was only twenty-four years old when his *Migration* series was featured in *Fortune* magazine. It was the first time that a major magazine featured the work of an African American artist, and it catapulted him into the spotlight. It was all very overwhelming for the young man, and he grappled to understand why he was accepted while others were not. Where were his peers? Lawrence felt isolated, alone, and confused.[4]

There is a parallel here with Jean-Michel Basquiat, who gained significant attention as a Black artist and incorporated many themes of race into his work, though Lawrence was born decades earlier than Basquiat and they faced unique struggles. Art historian Regenia A. Perry notes that Lawrence was "one of the few painters of his generation who grew up in a Black community, was taught primarily by Black artists, and was influenced by Black people."[5] Both Basquiat and Lawrence struggled with being seen as the sole artistic voice for the Black experience, Basquiat once lamenting that he had been tokenized as a "mascot."[6] Their experience reflects that of many other prominent African Americans; Jackie Robinson and Langston Hughes are two additional examples of Black men during Lawrence's time also expected to excel as "race representatives," despite the complex dynamics of racism in the country.[7] So, on the one hand, Lawrence was making great strides for himself as an artist, as well as raising awareness about key cultural experiences and issues. **On the other hand, he felt his success in some ways separated him from the community he sought to represent**.

In the asylum, Jacob Lawrence painted his fellow patients, and also the emotional ups and downs he went through personally, from the flaws he saw in the system there (such as too much sedation of patients), to the things that worked well for him (such as art therapy sessions). He spent nine months institutionalized and, upon his release, the *Hospital* series garnered a lot of attention. A mostly white art world said that it was his best work. *Ebony* magazine has questioned whether this was subtle racism; did the critics like the work better because it reflected a white experience, even if it was that of people in a mental hospital?[8]

Regardless of these questions, the hospital stay helped Lawrence, who stated that the therapeutic guidance he received there was one of the most meaningful experiences of his life. He also credited his wife, painter Gwendolyn Knight, for her unwavering support during his stay.[9] With depression, people might experience a single depressive period, or they might suffer from chronic relapse. In Lawrence's case, he spent approximately nine months in inpatient treatment, before and after which he never seemed to have another major depressive period.

Lawrence was institutionalized alongside people in varied states of well-being and distress, coping with myriad mental health issues and their symptoms, and he depicted them in his paintings. There was something he noted about his fellow patients that was similar to his subjects from the outside world: "These people are facing a struggle inside themselves that is just as intense as that of the Freedom Fighters I've painted."[10] In this way, his *Hospital* series is perhaps not that far a departure from his other work. The paintings are still concerned with **marginalized and stigmatized people working their way through personal and societal challenges.**

The *Hospital* series gives us insight into Lawrence's experience personally, as well as into how this particular institution functioned at that time in history. It also reveals that Lawrence was not without conflict regarding the patients' treatment. For example, his piece *Sedation* reflects upon one of the most widely debated aspects of mental health treatment: medication. *Sedation* depicts a group of seven people, in slumped positions, wearing what look like pajamas or scrubs, standing in a circle around a tray. The tray holds seven brightly colored pills that make up the majority of the painting's focus. It's as though the people are an afterthought—the medication is what matters here. The patients are neither reaching for the medication nor backing away. Instead, they just stand there resigned, perhaps already too sedated to care. Their hair is matted and their heads hang down, either a symptom of depression, a side effect of the sedatives, or the result of days of repetitive drudgery in an institution. As author Morgan Hampton describes:

> *Sedation* poses an important question: is it mental illness, or the treatment of mental illness that truly subdues you? These patients . . . gather around their enclosed pills with both a willingness and a reluctance to take them. It's a sad dichotomy. We don't see what choice they end up making, but it's important to note that . . . the pills residing behind glass represent a barrier that these patients have to cross if they choose to take [them].[11]

There's a question in this painting about whether the problem is the illness or the "cure." Sometimes medication helps, sometimes it makes things worse, and sometimes it's just one part of a total solution.

Lawrence's piece *Creative Therapy* offers a more positive take on what can happen in the asylum, particularly in terms of healing treatment. It depicts the artist participating in an art therapy group led by a psychiatrist, in which he explored different aspects of his art, using color and perspective in new ways to explore his emotions. Art does have therapeutic value, and when artists are allowed to use it in therapy, it can make all the difference in whether their creative impulse shrivels or thrives. For Lawrence, it was a helpful means of self-expression. His hospital therapist, Dr. Emmanuel Klein, believed that despite the persistent myth that art comes from mental anguish, it actually derives from "the healthiest part of the personality."[12] This returns us to the ongoing historical debate about "madness and genius." On one side are the people who believe that the two are inextricably linked, that the most-innovative creative work comes from the same place as mental health challenges. This doctor is on the other side of the argument, with the belief that it is the healthy part of the brain or soul that creates, not the part struggling with psychopathology. As with most questions in this book, the "truth" is probably somewhere in the middle, and much more individual than an either/or perspective allows.

On the spectrum of mental health challenges, Lawrence was generally healthy, with the exception of one dark period, and was able to paint prolifically for years after. On the spectrum of artistic impulse, he was clearly moved to create, remaining inspired while institutionalized for his depression and even finding solace in documenting his hospitalization. His experience is a testament to using art as a tool to better understand one's own life experience, and to connect to others who may be going through similar ordeals.

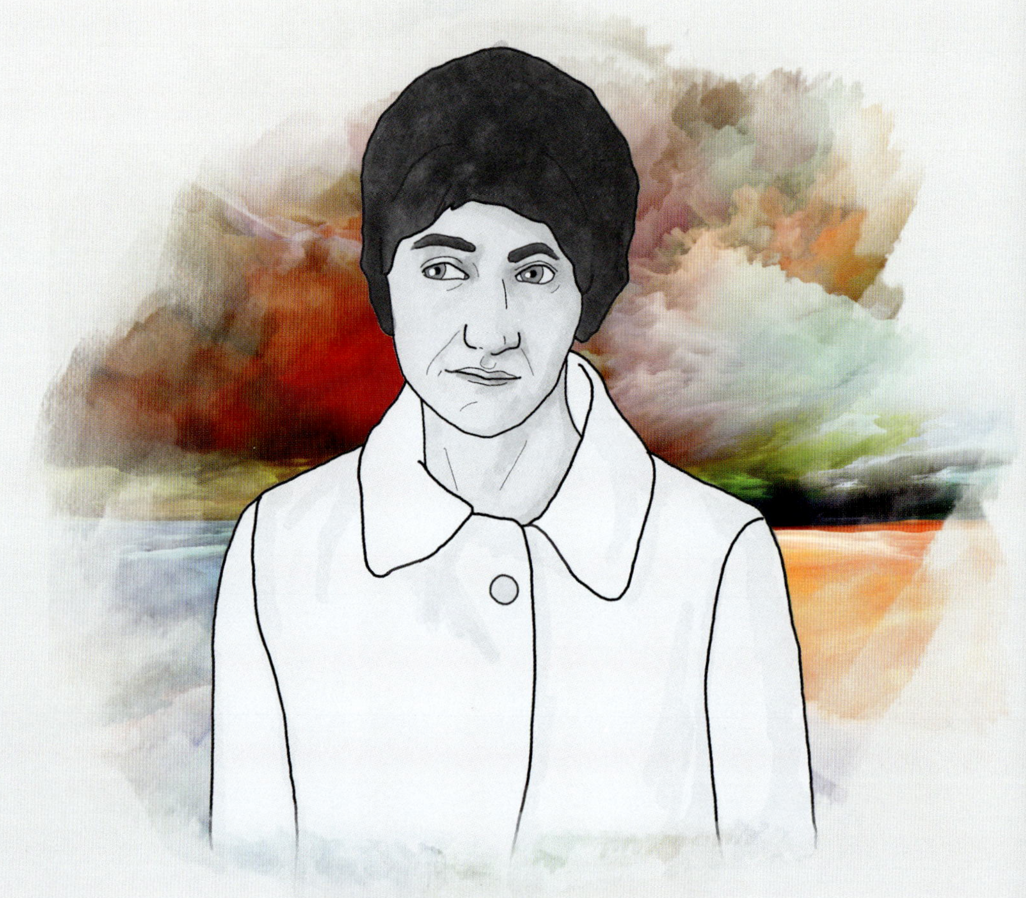

DIANE ARBUS

(March 14, 1923–July 26, 1971)

Most people go through life dreading they'll have a traumatic experience. Freaks were born with their trauma. They've already passed their test in life.

—DIANE ARBUS[1]

Diane Arbus is widely known as the photographer who photographed "freaks," the unfortunate terminology she uses to refer to a broad spectrum of people, from so-called circus freaks ("Siamese twins," giants, little people) to those who simply didn't fit into society's norms of the time (the LGBTQAI+ community, nudists, people with disabilities). Essentially, a freak was anyone who was "different." Arbus's work is controversial, but it undoubtedly paved the way for countless artists who came after her, including Nan Goldin and Robert Mapplethorpe.

When people talk about the photography of Diane Arbus, they tend to overemphasize the "freakishness" of her subjects. Some also oversimplify Arbus by defining her as a highly sexual woman who regularly put her own safety and even life at risk by visiting dangerous areas to photograph the people there. This is arguable. On one hand, it may simply reflect society's often-puritanical norms and expectations of women, especially women such as Arbus who came from "proper" (well-to-do) backgrounds. She was known to sometimes have sex with her subjects, once even participating in an orgy; this perhaps makes her sexually adventurous, but it doesn't necessarily mean that she had any kind of problem. Demeaning her sexual energy and calling the areas she visited "dangerous" could reflect the conventions of the time more than anything else.[2]

That said, if we imagine that these claims of risky behavior have some validity (there are accounts where she said herself that she was afraid of the places she went, although whether she was simply anxious or truly fearful for her life is up for debate), then we can also consider the role that Arbus's mental health played in these choices. We know that Arbus suffered from depression, and it is possible that it was **bipolar depression**—that pushing herself to create in dangerous situations was part of a manic phase. Biographer William Todd Shultz quotes a letter Arbus wrote in 1968 describing extreme ups and downs where she is "breathless with excitement," and then, just as quickly, her "energy . . . just leaks out,"[3] a description that might indicate **rapid cycling bipolar depression**. Moreover, sexual risk-taking can also occur in the manic phases of bipolar depression, although it's challenging to judge what exactly is "risk-taking" versus normal sexual expression that is being stigmatized. All of that said, experts generally concur that she was more likely bipolar than unipolar. People with bipolar depression often get misdiagnosed with major depression, particularly if they seek treatment during depressive periods, rather than while manic. If it's true that she lived with unipolar depression and if it's true that she was unusually promiscuous (again, taken with a grain of salt) and that she pursued her art in situations that felt dangerous to her, there could be another explanation: perhaps Arbus was simply trying to feel something.

Depression rips feeling away from you, leaving you numb or empty. You may experience thoughts of hopelessness and worthlessness and lack passion or interest. But there is a part of humanity that yearns to thrive. Often, that part will speak up and push someone to try to feel something, anything at all. **Everyday experiences might have been too banal to break through her despondency.** Perhaps her attraction to sex and danger, if not explained by normal human curiosity or by bipolar mania, simply demonstrates a drive to feel alive. Several people have noted that Arbus had an almost compulsive need to take photographs. As journalist Jenna Ross put it, "Hunting down subjects on the fringes of society was her drug, and she was constantly pursuing the high."[4]

Sigmund Freud, whose theories have many problems to consider but who nevertheless played a key role in the history of psychology, posited that we have two drives: Eros, the sexual drive of life, and Thanatos, the death drive.[5] One could argue that working through her depression, Arbus was attempting to thwart one so the other could thrive. Biographer Arthur Lubow writes of Arbus's recollection being a girl at summer camp: when all of the other girls were bitten by leeches, she was disappointed she was not: "She complained that she had rarely felt anything in her entire life. She was untouched by the ordinary joys and pains that make people feel alive. This was her prison."[6] Lubow also notes that in Arbus's search for the "promise of direct feeling," she found that "childbirth and menstruation were two of the only experiences that had provided her with the sense of being connected, almost the sole experiences that had bestowed upon her a twinge of joy."[7]

Despite this admitted numbness to joy and pain, Diane Arbus had a striking ability to pull the drama out of any situation and illuminate it through portrait photography. One of her most famous photographs, *Child with a toy hand grenade in Central Park, NYC*, is exemplary of this skill. The photograph is a powerful image of a knobby-kneed, dirt-stained boy holding a plastic grenade in the park, his mouth set into a grim, serious expression and his eyes bursting wildly out from the image. Author Deborah Nelson explains how this photograph was number eight in a set of eleven that Diane took of the boy, none of which were particularly remarkable, except for this one.[8] In all of the other images, he looks like a normal, happy little boy playing in the park. In the photo she chose to print and publish, he looks entirely different. Perhaps this wildness reflects his true self, and Arbus was able to capture it in only one frame. Or perhaps the boy is a symbol, representative of a certain excitement or intensity Arbus was seeking from life and from the people that she encountered.

Arbus's body of work has often been pathologized because of her biography. As *New York Times* writer Lyle Rexer attests, her work "cannot be disentangled from the tragedy of her depression and death."[9] But fellow *New York Times* book critic Parul Seghal complains that Arbus "receives diagnoses in place of critical analyses."[10] While not overstating the effect that Arbus's mental health had on her artistry, it is interesting to explore how her life story intersects with her creative choices. Arbus had documented periods of depression as early as age eleven. Her mother also suffered from depression, once suffering a breakdown so severe she was unable to function for many months. From this we might conclude that there may have been a genetic predisposition or component of intergenerational trauma to her condition. Lubow reports that teachers were concerned about her depression, and that she was described as emotionally fragile. Her early photographs from this time were as "wispy and frail" as she was—a blurred and out-of-focus image of a balloon floating away, for example.[11] Though we must be cautious of moralizing, we also can't ignore the issue of sex as it applies to Diane Arbus, because it plays a prominent role in her work and is likely relevant to her early childhood depression. In Lubow's 2016 biography, he revealed the shocking confession that not only had Diane likely had an incestuous relationship with her brother when she was a child, but that they had resumed the affair as adults.[12] We can only guess at the sexual trauma and unhealthful dynamics that may have been at play in that relationship.

Sexuality is complicated to define. But when a family story involves incestuous relationships, there is, at the very least, an extreme lack of boundaries. Often, when one doesn't learn boundaries in their childhood home, it becomes difficult to embody them later in life. This could speak to Diane's attitude toward sexual relationships, which Alex Mar says "contributed to the instability of her life, confused some of her friendships (both social and professional), and possibly made her sick."[13]

Diane did photograph sexual subjects: she went to swingers' parties, sex clubs, and other places where she could photograph people during sex acts. Although she's been called promiscuous, it's also important to remember that this was the era of the sexual revolution, and Arbus was participating in and documenting an important cultural moment. Art is often a way that individuals come to better understand themselves; it is a form of catharsis, and her interest in photographing sex could perhaps have come from her own struggle to understand its role in her own life, both considering the confused relationships of her childhood, and within the greater historical context.

Sex can also be an act of self-affirmation. Like many artists and people with mental health issues, Arbus struggled throughout her life to understand her own identity. She had been born into wealth, despite the Great Depression affecting so many other families around her, a fact that always made her feel guilty.[14] That she was drawn to photograph "freaks" and outsiders, and to connect with them through sex, might have been reflective of "a deeper desire to remake herself and to be accepted as a self-styled outsider," as journalist Sean O'Hagan writes.[15] Seduction of her portrait subjects (both artistically and sexually) may have been a way to establish herself in the world.[16] People in her life noticed this lack in Arbus of a defined sense of self and have posited that perhaps she also sought fame as a means of defining her self-worth.[17]

If we see Arbus's art as a fight to understand herself and to stave off the numbness of depression, then perhaps we can learn the most from her last series of photographs, which she started in 1969 and left incomplete when she died in 1971. The *Untitled* series consists of photos she took at a residential facility for individuals with developmental disabilities. She photographed the women residents, commenting to her daughter that they looked the same age as her but behaved like children.[18] Writer Jacquie Palumbo reminds us that at this point in history, the developmentally disabled were put into the same category as those with mental health issues such as schizophrenia or depression.[19] What can we make of Diane's intense focus on photographing this population during a time when she must have been struggling with her own mental health? Did she see herself reflected in the faces of those she photographed at the institution? Did it make her think about her own childhood?

In the 1972 documentary about Arbus's life, titled *Masters of Photography: Diane Arbus*, she is quoted as saying that people have an actual self and an intended self, and that she liked to capture the gap between the two.[20] She wanted to photograph a person disarmed, when the way in which someone tries to present themselves to the world fades and their internal or "true" self comes through. Of course, as the photographer she has the artistic liberty to determine what she portrays as a person's "true" self. For example, in *Child with a toy hand grenade in Central Park, NYC*, she apparently determined that the grim, frustrated face of the boy was most accurate to his true self, "truer" in some way than the silly, playful child in the other photos that she opted not to publish. For a long time, people criticized this photograph, accusing Arbus, with her fascination with "freaks," of cherry-picking the shots that made her subjects look the strangest. However, when Arthur Lubow interviewed the child in the photograph, Colin Wood, as an adult, Wood said that Arbus had captured exactly what he was feeling at the time. His parents were divorcing, and he was an angry, upset kid, prepared to "pull the pin" on a grenade.[21] Arbus saw humans as having at least three faces—the one they show to the world, the one they really are, and the one in between. **Perhaps her attention to multiplicity in her photographs was a way for her to reconcile her own fragmentation, or the gaps in her self-understanding.**

Biographer Patricia Bosworth describes that Arbus continued to struggle with depression throughout the 1960s. By this time, she had been diagnosed with hepatitis and blamed her depressive symptoms on the disease, the most prevalent being extreme exhaustion.[22] Having had a bad reaction to medication in the past (a drug called Vivactil made her depression worse and caused her anxiety), she refused to try the antipsychotic drugs that were recommended by her doctor. Instead, she opted for therapy, attending weekly sessions for two years leading up to her death. Despite these efforts to get better, Arbus died on July 26, 1971, from an overdose of barbiturates in combination with slitting her wrists, the same combination of methods by which Mark Rothko died just one year prior.

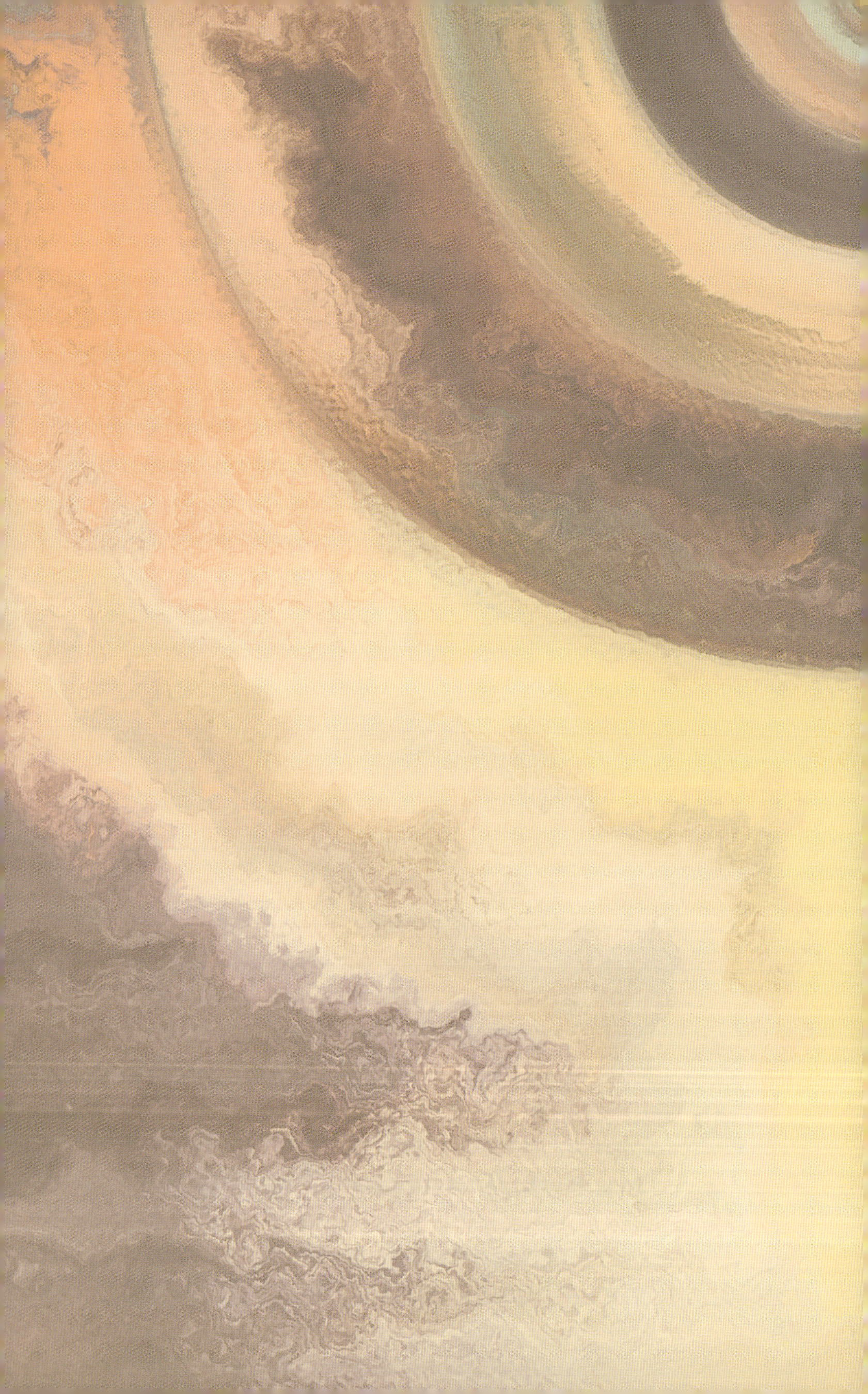

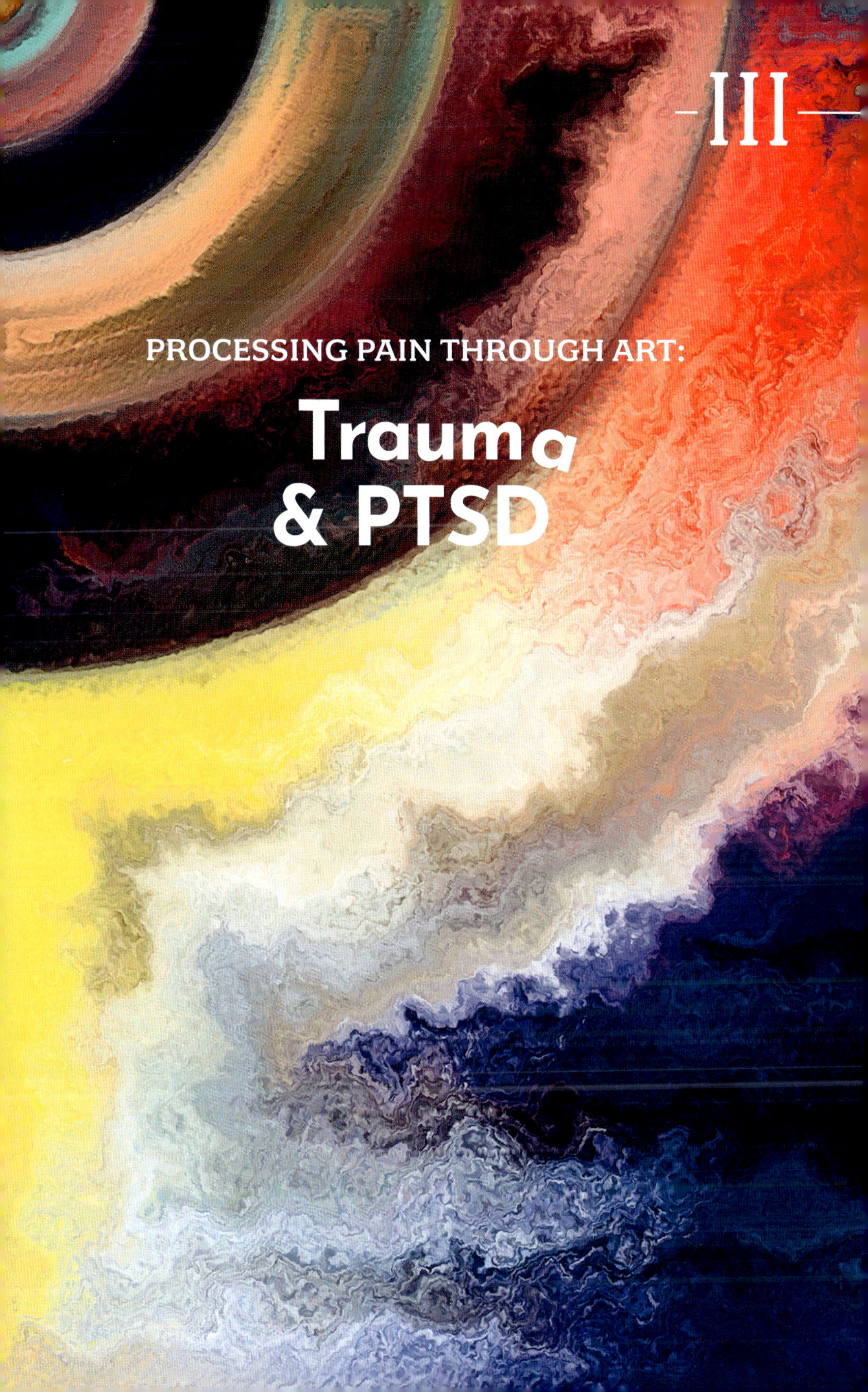

—III—

PROCESSING PAIN THROUGH ART:

Trauma & PTSD

Through the stories that we've already explored, we can see that there's a **link between trauma and mental health challenges**, one that the field of psychology continues working to understand. At the foundation, we know that mental health, and the way that it plays out in a person's life, consists of some combination of nature and nurture. A person has a certain proclivity toward mental health issues due to their genetics, but whether and how those issues get activated is deeply influenced with life experiences, including any traumatizing event that may occur, especially during the developmental years of childhood and early adulthood.

It's a complicated interplay of internal and external factors.

When trauma happens, art making is often a way for an artist to work through that experience. In this section we will explore the ways in which art emerges from trauma, by looking at the lives of artists who have experienced it, and the work they subsequently created.

WHAT IS TRAUMA?

Works of art always spring from those who have faced the danger, gone to the very end of experience, to the point where no human being can go.

–RAINER MARIE RILKE[1]

Historically, trauma as a mental health condition was most strongly associated with veterans returning from war who were diagnosed with posttraumatic stress disorder (previously called, among other names, shell shock). Over time, the field of psychology has come to recognize that there are many different types of traumas. Moreover, we have learned that there is a wide range of reactions to it that are not limited to PTSD.

Additionally, we have come to see that many mental health issues initially diagnosed alone are actually rooted in traumatic experience.

So, what is trauma? **Trauma is a response to an event, or a series of events, that one finds extremely distressing. People who experience trauma lose their sense of self, feel challenged in coping with daily life, and often have difficulty experiencing their emotions clearly, either becoming numb or becoming hypersensitive and easily overwhelmed.** It can be something that happens to you, something you witness, or something that happens around you. For example, growing up in a home where there is domestic violence is traumatic, whether or not you are the one physically victimized. The experience of poverty or sociopolitical instability in your country can be traumatic. Single traumatic events include such things as a serious car accident, sexual assault, natural disasters, or the loss of a loved one.

After a trauma, you might receive a diagnosis of PTSD or depression, which remain stigmatized conditions despite increased awareness in the twenty-first century. But there's another way of looking at our reactions to these events. In an article that applies feminist theory to trauma and "psychiatric disability," Andrea Nickl posits that mental health symptoms, such as depression, are the body's natural, normal, and healthful reaction to trauma.[2] She compares this to a physical injury—when the body is harmed, it needs time to heal. You may limp or scar. It's perfectly normal. We don't stigmatize people for needing to rest a broken leg, nor should we fault them for having to rest their mind after experiencing something terrible.

In this section, we'll look at some artists whose lives are characterized by different types of trauma. In some cases they have a mental health diagnosis that could occasion inclusion in our sections on depression or schizophrenia, which emphasizes the overlap between trauma and other mental health issues. Frida Kahlo, for example, had a diagnosis of depression but is included here because of the many traumas in her life. In other instances, such as with Jean-Michel Basquiat, there was no formal diagnosis, but we can clearly see the impact of traumatic childhood events on the artist. We will keep in mind our spectrum of interrelated factors: nature and nurture, era and culture, and diagnosis and treatment will all have an impact on our subjects' mental health and creativity.

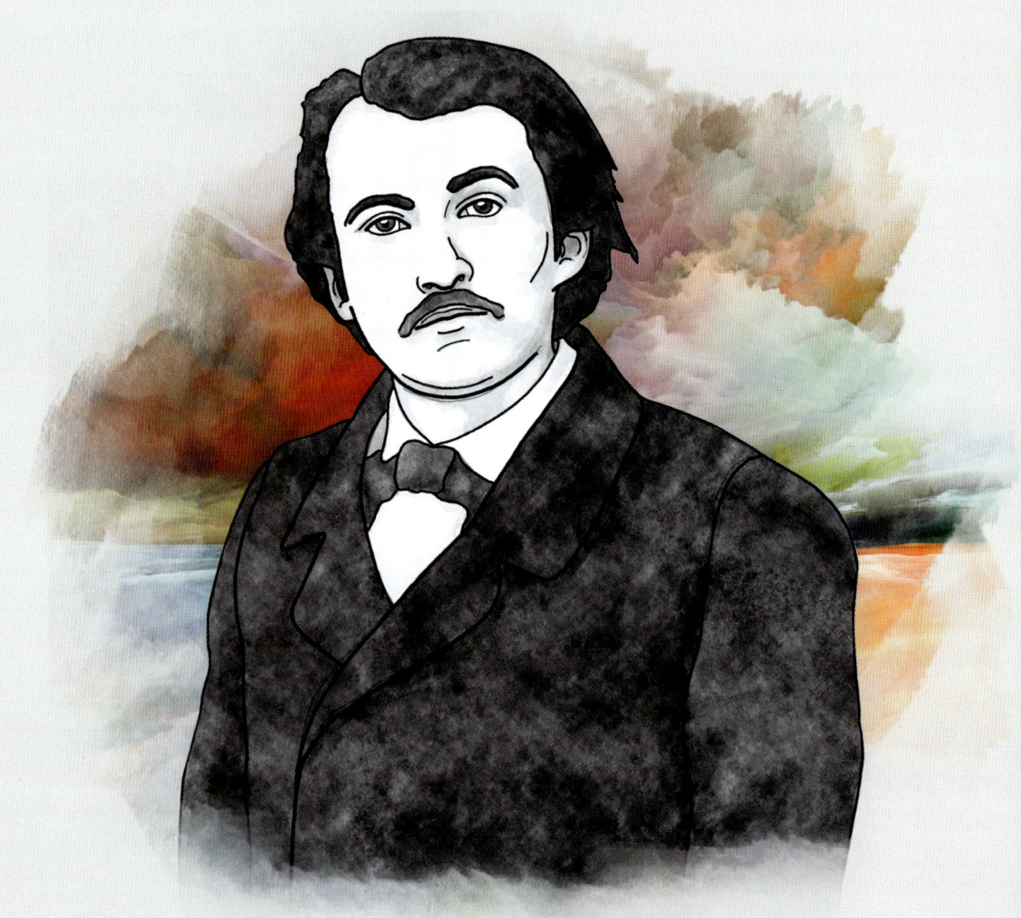

Gustave Doré

(January 6, 1832–January 23, 1883)

I am always, dear friend, in the shadow of an awful solitude, which I live in since so long a time . . . nothing consoles me; for I am alone, alone, alone . . . life is but a cursed and absurd thing.

–GUSTAVE DORÉ[1]

Gustave Doré is one of the first artists whom author and art historian Linda Nochlin draws attention to in her groundbreaking book *Misère: The Visual Representation of Misery in the 19th Century*, about **"misère," a form of widespread cultural depression.** Doré provides an excellent example of how depression can be both a personal challenge and societal one felt by a large percentage of the population during certain times in history. Misère is poverty-induced depression that has an impact on people living in industrial nations when they have to coexist beside great wealth. With the middle class eroding in our own modern-day United States, it's important for Americans today to look at this type of depression, and to examine the role it played in history (including art history), in order to perhaps better understand our own current reality.

When there is a large gap in wealth, it is normal for those at the bottom of the system to feel rage and frustration at the inequity. When a disadvantaged financial status combines with issues of intersectionality (misogyny, racism, xenophobia, etc.), the individual (or group of individuals) might experience even-more-turbulent emotions. More than anything else, one can begin to feel both helpless and hopeless. That's misère—the burden of the unfairness of the world, and the understanding that the experience of poverty is a form of trauma. Today, research about communities with lack of access to basic resources has indicated that being impoverished can lead to a wide range of health issues, both physical and mental, that can linger for generations.[2]

Linda Nochlin explores this condition in depth through an art-historical lens in her book. Art has intersected with activism throughout much of history in order to raise awareness of such inequities, and Gustave Doré provides an excellent example for exploring this relationship.

Doré was an engraver and illustrator whose artwork was published in many important middle-to-late-nineteenth-century writings, including Dante's *Inferno*. He also did 180 engravings for an 1872 book called *London: A Pilgrimage*, which depicts the growing misère in England's capital city thanks to the riches of the Industrial Revolution, a period of technological advancement and economic growth that created wealth for some and disenfranchised many more. As Peter Ackroyd puts it in the introduction to a new edition of the book, "In the latter half of the nineteenth century London had become the wonder and the horror of the age."[3]

One of Doré's works that Nochlin points out as especially relevant to today is *Bulls-eye*. The artist uses light and shadow to dramatically capture the unfair distribution of power between policemen and a group of impoverished people. The officers wield bright lights while the poor citizens are stuck in their glare. It's a familiar issue—the misère of nineteenth-century London reflected in this work mirrors twenty-first-century conflicts that people of color and other oppressed groups face in regard to policing and prison today. *The River Bank—Under the Trees* is another pointed piece by Doré. It's a scene of people who are watching boat races; the wealthy under the trees are well dressed, delighting in the leisure of a picnic lunch. Above them, a group of poor people creep around in the trees, trying to get a good look at the spectacle from a crowded and uncomfortable position. The title of the piece indicates that we shouldn't even pay attention to them; the only people that matter are the beautiful and rich "under the trees."

Let's look at one more artwork that represents Doré's interest in the negative societal effects of modernization: *Over London—By Rail*. Nochlin describes this work, saying it "at once brings out the modernity of the great city and the dehumanizing mechanical repetitiveness that modern advances like the railroad bring to those who live in their shadow."[4] Of course, the railroad is no longer modern today. But you need only look at any major American city where luxury condo buildings loom over people experiencing homelessness to see that the misère that plagued nineteenth-century London remains relevant.

We experience societal problems both individually and collectively. Gustave Doré had his own struggles with depression (then called melancholy), while simultaneously existing in a time of great misère. His art reflects both, serving as social commentary and individual catharsis. Doré's own personal struggle with depression has frequently been linked to a history of rejection; although his work was well received in London, critics in Paris consistently turned their noses up at it. As such, Doré would often become despondent after periods of intense work. Biographer Blanche Roosevelt quotes the letters of his close friend Paul Dalloz, who emphasized that Doré's illustrations for Dante's *Inferno* were works of unparalleled genius for which he did not receive any acclaim. Dalloz's letter quotes Madame Doré, who describes her son as "mortified, humiliated, crushed, in despair" and recounts that he was unable to eat or sleep, which, as we know, are classic symptoms of depression. Dalloz posits that the combination of working so hard only to meet the ensuing rejection was simply too much for Doré to bear.[5]

One seemingly incongruous fact about Doré is that he was also described as having a happy and playful personality.[6] He was perhaps one of those people you would look at and say, "He doesn't *seem* depressed." There is a fallacy of what depression looks like from the outside that people often fall prey to. Someone can look as though they are doing perfectly well but be struggling intensely on the inside. Biographer Frank Henry Norton minimizes Doré's depression in this way, describing him as "joyousness of temperament" even late in life, and "only sometimes subject to fits of depression."[7] An 1874 magazine article better captures Doré's personality, noting that people who do comment on his depression describe it in dramatic, dark detail, and that perhaps it is the contrast between his "vein of grim and morbid pathos" and his "almost boyish freshness and bonhomie" that results in such dramatic portrayals of city life within his artwork.[8] Describing his illustrations for Poe's *The Raven* (which was his last work, published posthumously), Maria Popova writes, "Doré's engravings capture with piercing precision the heart of Poe's poem, that bewitching interplay between the light toward which we reach in the grip of longing and the darkness into which longing plunges the psyche when it becomes a nightmarish fixation."[9] This perhaps reflects the artist's struggle to appear content while experiencing inner turmoil, as well as the discordant experience of living in a society with extreme economic inequality.

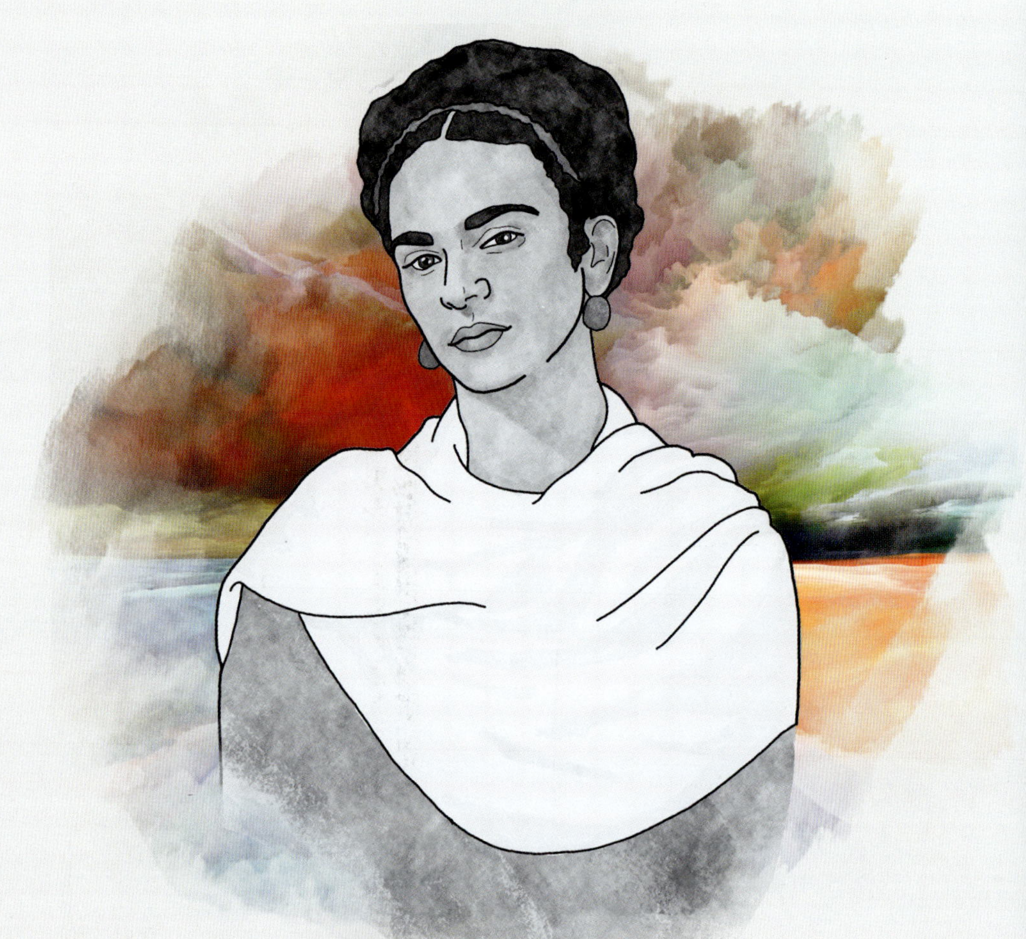

FRIDA KAHLO

(July 6, 1907–July 13, 1954)

> **Painting completed my life. I lost three children and a series of other things that would have fulfilled my horrible life. My painting took the place of all of this. I think work is the best.**
>
> **—FRIDA KAHLO[1]**

Frida Kahlo is perhaps one of the most interesting artists in history when it comes to exploring the links among trauma, mental health, and the power of artistic expression. Her life was marked by traumatic events, and her art chronicled those experiences through detailed self-portraiture. Although Kahlo referred to herself as "the great concealer," she agreed to undergo a series of psychological assessments late in her life that were incredibly revealing as to the effects of trauma on her psyche.[2]

Frida Kahlo was born into trauma. Her brother, the only son among her parents' five children, died shortly before she was born. After her birth, Kahlo's mother was mired in depression, and Frida was often left in the care of nannies.[3] She was, of course, too young to understand the rejection, and yet she absorbed the world as all babies do, internalizing the pain. Her mother's emotional withdrawal marked the first of many crises throughout her life.

Years later, upon her mother's death in 1932, Kahlo painted *My Birth*. In the painting, her mother is already dead while giving birth to her. Baby Frida, hanging half in and half out of the womb, also appears lifeless, her head resting limply upon blood-soaked sheets. This painting makes clear that Kahlo struggled throughout her life to make sense of her relationship with her mother, strained by feelings of abandonment caused by her mother's own grief and depression.

Frida's work, which is famously autobiographical, can't help but be of interest to those studying art as therapy. In fact, in 1947, Kahlo met Olga Campos, a psychology student who became her friend as well as her biographer. Campos was specifically interested in the psychology of creativity, and over the course of two years starting in 1949, Olga interviewed Kahlo about her life, and especially her childhood, while simultaneously conducting a series of psychological tests (including the Rorschach inkblot test and a word association test called the Bleuler-Jung test). Psychologist James Bridger Harris analyzed these tests in an early-twenty-first-century context, sharing the results in Salomon Grimberg's 2008 book *Frida Kahlo: Song of Herself*. In this summary, Harris diagnoses Frida with dysthymia (now called **persistent depressive disorder**), which is long-term chronic depression with periodic bouts of major depression. Harris also notes the influence of her chronic pain on her mental state and further argues that she qualifies for a diagnosis of "substance abuse in narcissistic personality."[4]

Beyond these diagnostic labels is Harris's assessment of Kahlo's **self-image** as it relates to her mental health. He describes that she tried throughout her life to establish her sense of self, which may explain her artistic obsession with **self-portraiture**. Although Harris doesn't specifically reference an attachment disorder, we know from decades of research in the field of psychology that attachment to the primary caregiver, usually the mother, plays a critical role in a person's development.[5] As a child, Kahlo could not see herself reflected in her mother's eyes but instead was met there with only emptiness. Kahlo spent the rest of her life attempting to stabilize her sense of self. Grimberg writes, "She grew up believing that she was not quite right the way she was, that to be more interesting, more desirable, she needed to become another person."[6]

Kahlo's early childhood trauma was, sadly, only the beginning of a life filled with tribulations. It has been well documented that the artist struggled with a variety of health issues.[7] She suffered from polio as a child, which caused deformities to one of her legs, exacerbating her sense of being different from others. At the same time, her illness gained her attention, particularly from her parents, ingraining into her a sense that people would be more likely to take care of her if she were sick than if she were able-bodied.[8] Of course, this isn't to say that she wanted to be sick or disabled, but to note that childhood experiences can create lasting patterns in the psyche. It can be lifelong work to understand and overcome those patterns.

Kahlo's most well-documented trauma is an accident that happened when she was eighteen. She was riding on the bus with her first serious boyfriend, Alejandro Gómez Arias, when the bus crashed, killing several people and severely injuring others, including Kahlo. She was impaled by a handrail from the bus, which pierced through her pelvis. This was the most severe of her many injuries from the crash, which included broken bones throughout her body. Kahlo was forced to spend months in bed during recovery; famously, this is when she began to paint.[9] She was her own first subject, using a mirror over the bed to see herself so that she could paint her image. The severe damage to her body occurred at a crucial point in adolescence, when Kahlo was discovering her sexuality and her sense of self as a woman; **her self-portraits from this time were undoubtedly a way to cope with the bodily trauma** and an attempt to gain insight into what kind of a woman she would become.

As is often the case, physical trauma coincided with emotional suffering throughout Kahlo's life. Arias, the boyfriend who was with her on the bus, had agreed to stay by her side throughout her recovery. But, having never been as in love with her as she had been with him, he promptly left for Europe after the accident, effectively abandoning Kahlo at her most vulnerable.[10] As we'll explore further in our chapter on Yayoi Kusama, there's a psychological theory called repetition compulsion in which we subconsciously reenact our early childhood and adolescent traumas, trying to get a different result in order to heal the original wound. Kahlo felt abandoned by her mother and would go on to choose relationships in which she would again have feelings of abandonment.

Undoubtedly, the most well known of these troubled relationships was her marriage to artist Diego Rivera. Their relationship was fraught from the start—Rivera had his first known affair one year into their marriage. Their first marriage was his third, and they stayed married for a decade, divorced, then remarried within a year. Rivera would never be faithful to her. In 1948, he asked for a second divorce to marry actress Maria Felix, a request Kahlo denied. The following year he wanted to marry Emma Hurtado, whom he ended up marrying after Kahlo's death.[11] The experience of betrayal from these requests for divorce was memorialized in a 1949 painting by Kahlo called *Diego and I*. It's a self-portrait of a teary Frida, with Diego sitting between her eyebrows, quite literally on her mind. We can contrast this to a painting with the same title she created in 1944, in which half of her face merges with half of Rivera's, creating a single entity. It is as though she never knew who she was without him. Although she would have affairs of her own, both with men and women, Kahlo spent most of her adult life trying to get confirmation of her self-worth from Rivera who, though twenty years her senior, was either unable or unwilling to provide her that assurance. In the foreword to Grimberg's *Song of Herself*, art historian Hayden Herrera writes that Kahlo "felt she was defective and ugly, feared abandonment, and needed other people's affirmation, especially that of her husband."[12]

The worst betrayal of all of Rivera's affairs was the relationship he had with her sister Cristina. Kahlo was so devastated by the news of their deception that she was unable to paint for several months.[13] Art had always been Kahlo's way of processing, but for a time it failed her. She experienced both depression and anxiety about her mental state, saying, "I can no longer continue in the very great state of sadness that I was in, because I was heading with large strides toward a neurasthenia of that horrible type that makes women turn into idiots."[14] Kahlo had internalized the idea of weak, sick women as "idiots," a troubling conclusion in light of her own physical handicaps. Moreover, she clearly feared the kind of immobility and lack of creative activity that came along with a neurasthenia diagnosis, due to the favored prescription of total bed rest. This fear motivated her to begin painting again, and when she did, her pain splashed onto the canvas.

Consider, for example, the 1938 painting *Passionately in Love*, also called *A Few Short Nips*, which was inspired by a newspaper article about a man who murdered his girlfriend in a bloody stabbing.[15] Author Celia Stahr argues that the work was truly about the hurt she experienced being rejected by Rivera, "Frida's own horrendous pain and the pain of all women." Stahr goes on to say, "The personal connection Frida felt with the painting is evident in the way she hung it in her studio and reworked it over the years . . . painting blood on the frame, putting stab marks in the frame, and leaving the knife sticking out of it."[16] Notably, the woman in the image is naked except for a shoe on her right foot, the foot of Frida's that was deformed from polio.

Another example from this time is *Memory, the Heart*, a painting that shows Kahlo with her heart pierced straight through, bleeding on the ground beside her. In this work she is dressed in European clothing, rather than the clothes expressing her Mexican heritage she usually painted in her self-portraits. Instead, her traditional clothes hang in the background of the painting. Once again we get the sense that Kahlo does not know who she is, and wants desperately to reinvent herself, or reclaim herself. After discovering the affair between her sister and Rivera, she "stopped wearing her Tehuana outfits and cut off the long black hair that Rivera loved."[17] We see this theme repeat years later in her 1939 painting *The Two Fridas*, painted after the couple's first divorce. The painting depicts a Frida in European dress holding hands with a Frida in traditional Mexican dress, the hearts of each Frida painfully exposed, the artery of one snipped through with scissors and bleeding.

As if all these life experiences were not traumatic enough, Kahlo also suffered the loss of three children. She had three abortions during a five-year span starting in 1929; the abortions were medically necessary due to her body's inability to carry a healthy baby to term. Kahlo likely had other miscarriages as well, since she was trying desperately to have a child.[18] She was surely struggling with the complex feelings that come along with infertility, as well as the grief of her miscarriages. To lose a baby at any stage is devastating; to have carried your child for three or four months only to lose them is highly traumatic, and this happened to her multiple times.

As you would expect, **Kahlo documented and processed these losses through her art.** Her 1932 drawing *Frida and the Abortion*, created after the loss of a second child, is a skillfully rendered and anatomically detailed self-portrait (Kahlo once hoped to become a medical illustrator) in which her nude body reveals a dead fetus in her transparent womb. This work also depicts the Mayan goddess of childbirth, Ixchel, in tears.[19] This work not only memorializes her trauma but is also one of the best examples of how art was critical to her sense of self and wellness. In the drawing, she may not be able to hold her now-dead child, but she does hold a heart-shaped painter's palette. Art was her baby, her mother, her lover, her constant companion.

Most likely due to these traumas, Kahlo struggled with alcohol as an adult. Her medical history notes that in 1939 she was drinking at least one bottle of cognac per day, attributed as a means of coping with her chronic pain and depression. By the following year, under the care of a new doctor in San Francisco, she was forbidden alcoholic beverages. Kahlo also reportedly may have had substance misuse issues with Seconal, which she took to sleep, and Demerol, which she took for pain.[20] Her chronic pain was also managed by meperidine and morphine, highly addictive drugs.[21] Kahlo's emotional pain was inextricable from her physical pain. Her physical condition kept worsening, and by 1944 she was prescribed "total rest and a steel corset,"[22] her fears of forced bed rest coming to fruition. It was necessary, though, since her neck and spine were in constant agony. Kahlo's mental health was noted as "general state: exhausted" in 1945, and then "very bad nervous agitation and great depression" the following year.[23]

During this time of forced bed rest, Kahlo painted *Without Hope*, the title of which clearly expresses how she felt about her situation. In the painting, Kahlo lies in bed, a huge easel atop her. However, instead of a canvas the easel holds a monstrosity: an oversized, grotesque bundle of dead animals dripping blood and flesh. The whole thing hovers ominously above Kahlo, whose arms appear pinned down beneath her blankets, as the carrion leaks directly into her mouth. By this time, due to her deteriorating mental and physical health, she was very thin and had no desire for food. Her doctor's prescription included force-feeding her a high-fat diet at regular intervals; the pureed food was funneled into her every two hours, a process she detested.[24] In the background of the painting is a beautiful but deserted Mexican landscape, the sun shining almost painfully bright and the moon hanging on the opposite side, perhaps indicating that from her bed the artist could not tell if it was day or night. The sun and moon also have powerful symbolic meaning in Aztec mythology, the sun representing human sacrifice and the moon womanhood.[25] On the back Kahlo inscribed, "Not the least hope remains to me. . . . Everything moves in time with what the belly dictates."

Things only continued to get worse for Frida Kahlo. In 1949, after Rivera asked to divorce her for the second time, she attempted suicide by overdose. She wrote her suicide note on his legal divorce request papers, and one line read, "I will not paint again, nor walk, I want to die."[26] Despite this incident, and one another suicide attempt, Kahlo continued to create through these tragedies.

In 1953, just before a devastating leg amputation, she wrote to Diego Rivera, "I was already a maimed woman when I lost you, again, for the umpteenth time maybe, and still I survived. . . . I am not afraid of pain and you know it." She goes on, "I told you I've counted myself as incomplete for a long time, but why the fuck does everybody else need to know about it too? Now my fragmentation will be obvious for everyone to see, for you to see."[27] Kahlo had spent her entire life feeling incomplete, and this amputation was the final straw in her lifelong physical battle. She died the following year.

Frida Kahlo's artwork, however, lives on. In fact, Kahlo has grown only more popular throughout the years. In many ways, Kahlo laid herself bare through her artwork, and her honesty resonates with many people. In his psychological assessment, Harris writes, "No other artist of Kahlo's stature has been courageous enough to make herself as vulnerable."[28] Perhaps this is why so many can recognize a piece of themselves in her work.

In an interesting intersection of art history and medicine, Fernando Antelo, for the *AMA Journal of Ethics*, cites Kahlo's work as critically insightful for physicians who want to better understand their patients in pain. He writes, "Her paintings are a medium to visualize pain and the effect of pain on the human condition."[29] Antelo notes that her work can be used as a tool through which others can discuss their own experience, highlighting that "a New York psychologist uses Kahlo's artwork in therapy sessions to help women talk about their experiences of emotional and physical trauma such as infidelity, violence, and infertility."[30] Frida Kahlo's art was catharsis for her, a way to move through her trauma, so it is fitting of her legacy that it continues to serve as a catalyst for others' healing to this day.

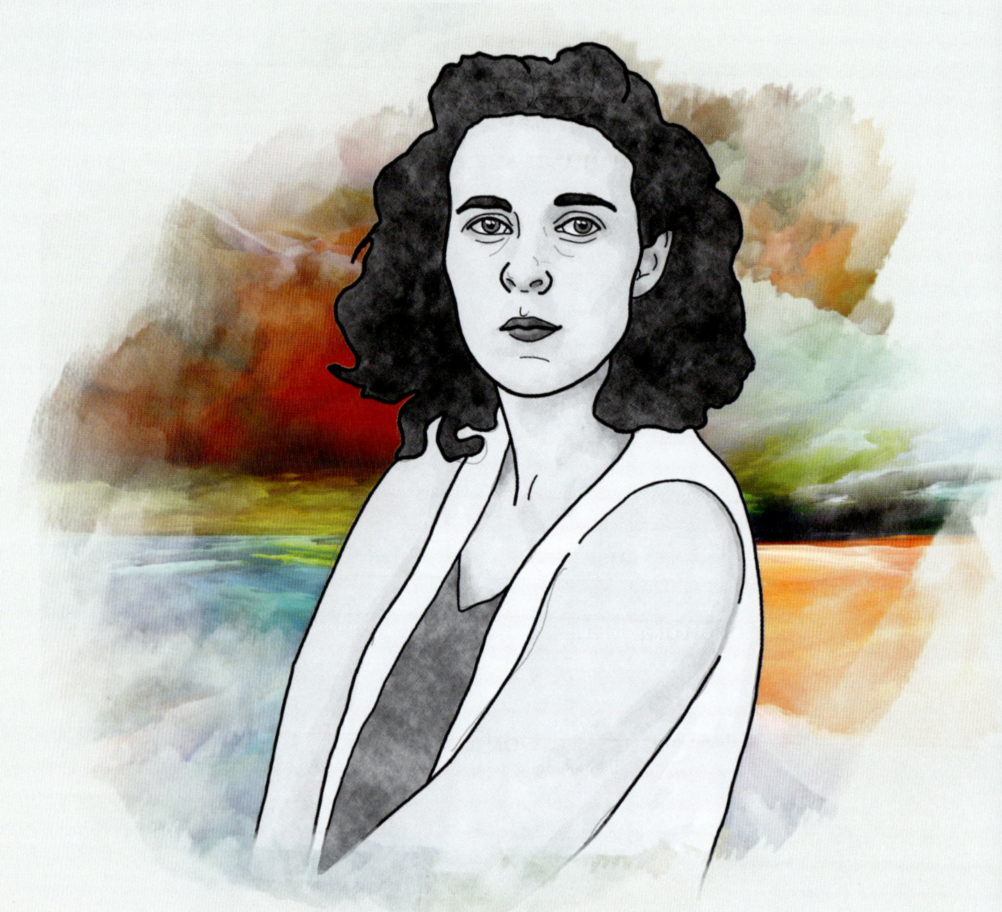

Leonora Carrington

(April 6, 1917–May 25, 2011)

Art is a magic which makes the hours melt away and even days dissolve into seconds.

–LEONORA CARRINGTON[1]

Surrealist painter and novelist Leonora Carrington experienced a psychotic episode as a result of various personal traumas and the sociocultural trauma of the Second World War. Always a dreamer, interested in probing the depths of her own mind, Carrington was able to channel her profoundly troubling experiences into a unique artistic vision. The result is a world of her own making—imagined creatures, places, and events that she may not have discovered within herself had it not been for this break with reality. In Carrington's case, we will again see how the **creative impulse is sometimes ignited by trauma, and how creating can help artists live through it.**

Carrington grew up in an aristocratic English home and was influenced by the folklore shared with her by her Irish grandmother and her Irish nanny.[2] Her education included a lot of music, art, and language, which was common for women of her socioeconomic status at the time. Carrington loved creating art, but she didn't want to draw the landscapes that "proper women" were expected to depict; she wanted to draw fairies, mystical worlds, and the fantastical expressions of her own imagination.[3]

Carrington was expelled from more than one school for "rebellious behavior" and odd daydreaming, "like fantasizing that she was a levitating saint."[4] Her parents expected her to marry rich and settle down, and they made her go through the London debutante season as an older teenager.[5] She loathed the experience and later wrote a short story about it called "The Debutante," in which a young woman asks a hyena to take her place at a ball. The hyena agrees and dresses in the debutante's clothes. However, the hyena realizes that her own face won't do, so she calls for the debutante's maid, devours her, and rips off her face to wear as a mask to the ball. Ultimately, the hyena also becomes irritated by the debutante scene—to the point that she eats off the maid's face she so recently acquired and flees the dance.[6] This is perhaps the first hint at Carrington's impulse for escapism, as well as a fragmented sense of self.

Many of Carrington's stories and paintings have multiple characters and unsettling imagery where animals, humans, and masks all merge together. Biographer Joanna Moorhead posits that "Carrington broke herself apart into different aspects of her being, and her bestiary therefore represents individual aspects of her self."[7] This type of fantastical imagery is characteristic of surrealist art. It also draws parallels to Jungian psychology, of which many of the surrealists were fans. Jung believed that we all have not only a personal inner self but also a collective unconscious, and that there are universal symbols that express that unconscious. Symbols, such as animals, hold deep meaning; in dreams they show up to give the conscious part of the psyche glimpses into what lies underneath. **The surrealist visual language would become useful for Carrington later in life, when she uses art to process her trauma.**

Carrington's parents ultimately agreed to let her study art in London, where she met artist Max Ernst.[8] They began a relationship together despite their nearly thirty-year age gap, and the fact that he was already married.[9] They became a couple and were active members of the surrealist movement, a group that consisted mostly of male artists who saw women as subject matter for their own art. Carrington actively rejected the idea that she was there to inspire the men around her, saying, "I didn't have time to be a muse. I was too busy rebelling against my family and learning to be an artist."[10]

Carrington's ability to reimagine her role as a woman in society is directly connected to the events of World War II, the trauma of which also played a key role in her life, work, and mental health. Ernst, who was German, was arrested by the Nazis, who interned him in a concentration camp, in large part because of his artwork, which they considered "degenerate."[11] Carrington, not knowing whether or not he would ever return, was left alone in their countryside home as her friends fled France to escape the war.[12]

At this time Carrington began to develop odd behavior, including days-long fasting and obsessive exercise.[13] She got thinner and thinner and tried to cleanse herself by vomiting—all behavior suggestive of an **eating disorder**.[14] Food often plays a role in mental health challenges. In addition to eating disorders, people may eat too much or too little due to depression and anxiety, or they may develop food-related phobias. Carrington's mind began to deteriorate along with her body. The combined trauma of the war and losing Ernst to imprisonment led to her mental breakdown at the young age of twenty-three.[15] Worried about Carrington's declining mental health as the war progressed, fellow artist Catherine Yarrow arrived and encouraged her friend to get out of France.

Yarrow and Carrington set off to Spain together. Surrounded by the devastation of war, Carrington's mental health became increasingly worse throughout the journey.[16] Once during the trip, the car's brakes jammed and she believed that she and the car were one—that *she* was jammed and had caused the trouble with the brakes.[17] Carrington explains, "This was the first stage of my identification with the external world," meaning **a blurring of the boundaries between herself and the world around her**.[18] Writing of her arrival in Spain, Carrington says she felt "choked by the dead" and describes having delusions.[19] She writes of her emotional state at the time:

> In the political confusion and the torrid heat, I convinced myself that Madrid was the world's stomach and that I had been chosen for the task of restoring this digestive organ to health. I believed that all anguish had accumulated in me and would dissolve in the end, and this explained to me the force of my emotions. I believed that I was capable of bearing this dreadful weight and of drawing from it a solution for the world.[20]

This intense grandiosity, paired with her various odd behaviors, all were evidence of her decline into psychotic mental illness.[21] Carrington manifested both mental and physical health symptoms, including "exasperated nerves," "an inability to walk straight," communicating with animals and nature instead of humans, and "paralyzing anguish."[22] Later in her life, she made it clear that this experience was indeed the direct result of trauma, writing, "I'd suffered so much when Max was taken away to the camp, I entered a catatonic state, and I was no longer suffering in an ordinary human dimension."[23]

Carrington felt at times as if she was various animals, and at other times as if she was the entire universe. She had always been fanciful, representing herself as different animals in her art, but this was beyond a simple product of imagination or Jungian exploration of the collective unconscious. Carrington was truly unable to separate reality from delusion. Further compounding her distress, during this time she reports experiencing a sexual assault. After acting erratically at the British embassy in Madrid, she was placed in the Santander Mental Asylum. She recalls being tricked into going to the hospital: "On the way, I was given Luminal three times and an injection in the spine: systemic anaesthesia. And I was handed over like a cadaver to Dr. Morales."[24]

In the asylum, Carrington was given barbiturates as well as cardiazol, an alternative to electroshock therapy, which had horrifying side effects but was a common treatment for psychosis.[25] A psychiatric review of the drug describes it as inducing "seizures strong enough to fracture vertebrae and stop the heart."[26] Carrington's physical heart didn't stop, but the torturous treatment certainly had a detrimental effect on her soul. Like Alice Neel, she may have needed help for her condition, but she hated everything about the asylum.

Later, she would write about the traumatic experience of institutionalization in her memoir *Down Below*. Writing it was painful for her, but she did it anyway and, in doing so, gave the world terrific insight into the maltreatment of women in asylums.[27] (Though it should be noted that many professionals and researchers have dismissed the legitimacy of her claims of horror as products of a fantastical imagination, perhaps due to the nature of surrealism.)[28]

In addition to the medication-induced seizures, Carrington recalls "hallucinating naked and strapped to a bed, as she lay in her own feces" and describes feeling as though she were dead.[29] She was "repeatedly stripped and bound, prodded and penetrated, forced against her will to submit to invasive treatments."[30] Like Frida Kahlo, she was force-fed, and she hated being constantly observed through the glass.[31] One of the most violent "treatments" they forced her to endure was when doctors induced abscesses in her thighs, specifically to prevent her from walking.[32] Between these injuries and the barbiturates, she was effectively immobilized.

On top of these traumatic "treatments," Carrington admits to seducing one of her doctors, who was only happy to engage in the relationship.[33] This would be inappropriate and unethical in any context but is particularly vile given the power dynamics of institutionalization and her recent assault. **Sexual-assault survivors**

often grapple with mixed feelings, including undue guilt. Carrington's guilt was compounded by the horrors of World War II, which had sent her to the asylum in the first place. She more or less accepted the maltreatment in the asylum, not only because she felt powerless but also because she felt that they were "purifying tortures" that she, as "a Celtic and Saxon Aryan, was undergoing . . . to avenge the Jews for the persecutions they were being subjected to."[34] Gustave Doré experienced individual depression in the context of much-broader social malaise; here, we see Carrington's mental health impacted not only by personal traumas, but also by the trauma of war.

Carrington's mental health did ultimately improve, but it is unclear whether that was because of or in spite of her treatment in the asylum.[35] She did say the experience brought her "clarity and power of mind," but there is no doubt that her journey to health was a traumatic one, and that her traumas continued to influence her life choices.[36] Peggy Guggenheim (who was Max Ernst's partner after Carrington) noted that the artist always seemed to seek father figures, especially after the asylum, positing that she did so "to give her some stability and prevent her from going mad again."[37] Like we'll see with Jean-Michele Basquiat's relationship with Andy Warhol, this is the theory of **repetition compulsion** again, wherein people try subconsciously to repeat early flawed relationships in an effort to heal childhood wounds. Leonora didn't like to talk about her childhood, but she did once say that her father was more like a mafioso than anything else.[38]

Carrington moved to Mexico in 1942 and thrived there, exhibiting her work, publishing her writing, and marrying the love of her life, Emerico Weisz.[39] Weisz and Carrington raised two children in a relatively happy marriage, staying married for more than fifty years.[40]

We often think of mental illness, particularly when it includes psychosis and delusions, as a lifelong struggle for the individual. But in some instances, a person has a single, specific breakdown, emerges from it, and doesn't suffer from such issues again. Like Jacob Lawrence, who had one depressive period during a time of high stress, Carrington experienced only this one major psychotic break. This is why, although some have tried to posthumously diagnose her as such, she doesn't meet the criteria for schizophrenia, since it is a lifelong condition. In her case, the traumas surrounding her experience during World War II triggered her collapse. Though it would be the only breakdown she would have, it is well documented thanks to her art. Carrington never forgot the terror of the experience and always feared that it could happen again.[41]

Writing and making visual art about her break certainly seemed to be therapeutic for Carrington as she grappled with her childhood and her later traumas. Of "The Debutante," for example, writer Selena Chambers notes, "She is both the debutante and the hyena, a past and present evaluation (and catharsis) of her new life at the time of the story's composition in 1937." This harkens back to Frida Kahlo's *Two Fridas* and the artist's ongoing search for identity. Channeling one's life experience, especially trauma, into a unique artistic expression is perhaps at the heart of many artists' creative impulse. Journalist Elaine Salkaln writes, "Leonora heroically internalized what she learned on that journey: she taps into it and comes back, not only making art out of the richness of her discoveries, but also showing how to balance the opposing forces within us."[42] For Carrington, the breakdown was a breakthrough.[43]

Whether she was writing or painting, Carrington captured something ineffable, magical, and universal, something that she may not have been able to access were it not for her forays into the darker places of the mind.

Body Image and Art

Much has been written about the negative mental health effects of the cultural pressure to look a certain way. Not only perpetuated by the media, but reinforced by society at large, and subsequently internalized on an individual level, beauty standards are pervasive, and negative body image has been linked to mental health issues like depression, anxiety, and eating disorders, especially in women and girls.[1] Art can be an extremely effective way to boost self-esteem and express anger, resentment, or frustration about the burden to be beautiful. Jenny Saville, for instance, rejects the idea that paintings should reflect an idealized fantasy of what nude women should look like, instead celebrating the beauty of individualism and focusing on so-called "flaws" like fat rolls, cellulite, and sagging skin in her monumental, flesh-filled canvases.[2]

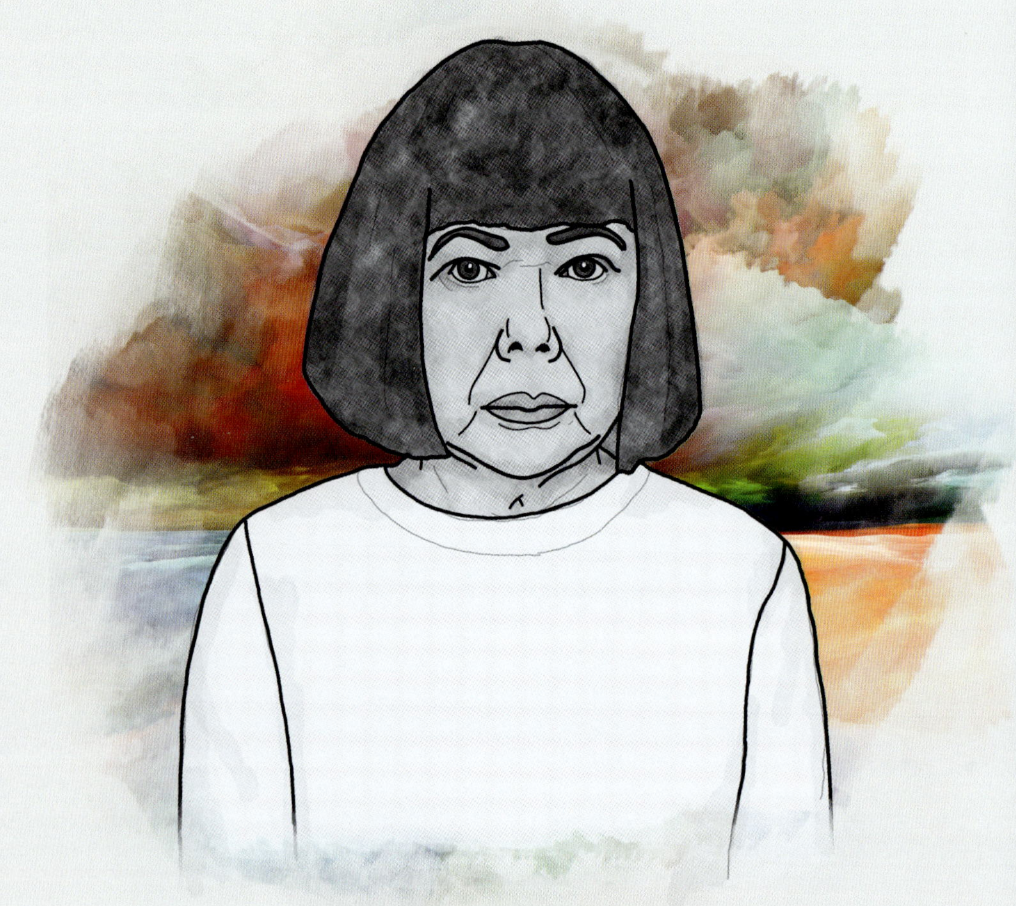

Yayoi Kusama

(b. March 22, 1929)

Anxiety felt like flickering flames in my bones.

–YAYOI KUSAMA[1]

Yayoi Kusama is the top-selling female artist in the world, and one of the world's best-known contemporary female artists. She has also lived in a mental health institution for more than half her life. Kusama is an excellent example to discuss when it comes to the relationship between a person's art and their mental health struggles, since not only is she still alive, but she has also been very open about the subject. Kusama explicitly states that making art helps her cope with her mental illness: "It's how I get away from my illness and escape the hallucinations. I call it psychosomatic art."[2]

If we look back at her early childhood, we can see that trauma may be at the root of Kusama's challenges. In the 2018 biographical documentary *Kusama: Infinity*, the artist's early years are described as persistently traumatic.[3] Kusama's parents' marriage was troubled. Her father even took her mother's maiden name as his own, apparently as a symbol of how impotent he felt in his own family. To gain some control or boost his self-esteem, he engaged in several extramarital affairs. Kusama reports that her mother would send her to spy on these affairs, and although we don't know the extent to which seeing her father in the throes of passion with strange women and reporting the scenes back to her mother influenced her mental health, we can guess that it wasn't easy for Kusama, who was already described as a "sensitive child."

At a young age, art was useful to Kusama as an outlet. However, she had to fight to continue making it, even as a child. Kusama tells one story of her mother, who did not support her art, coming up from behind her as she was drawing or painting to snatch the work out of her hands and destroy it.[4] Even today, eighty years later, Kusama works furiously fast and with a great sense of urgency, almost as though her body has never forgotten the panic of trying to get her art on the page before it could be stolen.

Trauma can be a single incident or a series of stressors. In the biographical documentary *Kusama: Infinity*, the artist describes another traumatic experience from childhood, although the event itself remains vague. She recalls a vision she had in a field as a child, where all the flowers started talking to her, and she felt as if she were disappearing into the endless landscape, consumed by them. This may have been a hallucination of some sort, or a warped-recollection traumatic event that her mind has since repressed. Whatever happened, the theme of flowers shows up throughout her life's work, as though she is continually processing the experience. Despite these distressing events in her childhood, Kusama did not hesitate to fight for her art as she grew older, and she became increasingly determined to make a career of it. Despite the lack of support from her parents, she eventually convinced them to let her go to art school. There, she learned about Georgia O'Keeffe's work and reached out to the older artist, seeking advice as a mentor (and, if we can speculate, perhaps the validation of a mother figure).[5] O'Keeffe encouraged Kusama to get herself to the United States, and in 1958 Yayoi did just that, moving to New York City to pursue her passions.

It was no easy path. She had to work hard to break into this men's world, particularly back in 1958. At the time, women artists were occasionally showing work at galleries alongside men, but never in solo exhibitions. Kusama also moved from Japan to America relatively soon after World War II. Between her marginalized identity as a Japanese person and the gender inequity of the time, the young artist had many biases working against her, and New York was a stressful environment. Yet, she remained impressively ambitious, saying of her intentions, "My goal was to create a new history of art in the United States."[6] Though determined, the anxiety of achieving her goals would soon begin to affect Kusama's mental well-being. She writes in her autobiography, "I found it all extremely stressful and was soon mired in neurosis."

Anyone who has experienced a **panic attack** will be familiar with the feeling of "the walls closing in." We can see Kusama directly confronting this symptom of anxiety in her artwork, perhaps in an attempt to gain control. In one interview she shares, "I'm obsessed with nets. They cover me, strangle me. They fascinate and haunt me."[7] She uses the word "panic" frequently to describe the feelings she has toward nets, similar to her childhood experience, and later artistic obsession, with flowers. Kusama described her *Infinity Nets* as paintings "without beginning, end, or center. The entire canvas would be occupied by [a] monochromatic net. This endless repetition caused a kind of dizzy, empty, hypnotic feeling."[8]

One harrowing experience Kusama retells is waking up one morning to see that the nets she had painted the night before were covering all the windows. When she reached out to touch them, the nets bled onto her hands and she went into a "full-blown panic attack." She checked herself into Bellevue Hospital repeatedly during this time, as she continued to endure severe panic attacks. Jo Applin describes how Kusama feels a breaking down of boundaries between herself and the space around her, a disassociation rooted in intense anxiety: "During these encounters Kusama feels herself flattening out and blurring into one continuous surface in which she, through a form of psychic camouflage, experiences herself as lost to the environment."[9] This seems to describe a form of **depersonalization**, which can be both a symptom of anxiety or other mental health issues, or a stand-alone diagnosis.

Institutionalization is not the only way in which formal psychology began to play a role in Kusama's life during her time in New York. She worried frequently about her mental health and decided to see a Freudian psychoanalyst.[10] Psychoanalysts from this school of thought, particularly at that time, were driven by the idea that current problems are informed by repressed trauma from childhood, particularly repressed sexual issues.

In her autobiography, Kusama says that she was "hide-in-the-closet-trembling" afraid of sex, most likely due to being forced to see her father engage in sexual activities as a child. She writes that she began making artistic penises, reproducing them again and again, as a form of "Psychosomatic Art" or **self-therapy**, hoping that the more she made them, the more she could get used to them and the less terrified she would be.[11] As we've discussed previously, repetition compulsion is the idea that we keep doing the same thing over and over again, trying to repeat, and thus repair, an early trauma. The repetition in Kusama's work throughout her life is like a visible representation of repetition compulsion. Kusama says, "Accumulation is the result of my obsession, and that philosophy is the main theme of my art." She also explicitly says, "My work is based on developing my psychological problems into art." She writes, "By continuously reproducing the forms of things that terrify me, I am able to suppress the fear."[12] She used this method with other things as well. For instance, she had a fear of food, particularly processed food, and so made macaroni sculptures in order to overcome her aversion.[13] Kusama calls this repetitive facing of her fears "obliteration," but in modern psychology it may be classified as a form of **exposure therapy**.

One of the most powerful examples of the idea of repetition to the point of oblivion is a 1967 film that Kusama made with experimental filmmaker Jud Yalkut, titled *Self-Obliteration*, in which she completely covers herself in dots until she disappears into them as they engulf the screen.[14] Jo Applin presents an interesting theory about this "self-obliteration," citing surrealist writer Roger Caillois, who describes a phenomenon called psychasthenia. Psychasthenia is "an anxious-obsessive compulsive condition" in which you merge with your surroundings in order to become invisible as a means to protect yourself from danger.[15] Kusama, painted in dots, camouflaged into a background of dots, could be practicing exactly the same thing. We also see this manifested in the descriptions of her hallucinations—the artist disappears into her surroundings as an act of self-preservation due to trauma.

In 1966, Yayoi Kusama attempted suicide by jumping from a window. Luckily, a bicycle broke her fall and she survived. After that she lived in darkness, remaining in bed for upward of a week at a time, her anxiety growing with an express "fear of the unknown" and growing increasingly depressed. Her poem and video installation *A Manhattan Suicide Addict* (which is also the name of her first autobiography) makes specific reference to her suicidal depression, with lines such as "Swallow antidepressants and it will be gone" and "Amidst the agony of flowers, the present never ends."[16] Kusama moved back to Japan in an attempt to change her environment, but the shame her community in Japan tried to foist upon her for flouting tradition, combined with the death of her father at this time, led to increasingly worse mental health issues. Back in her childhood environment, she was overcome by memories trauma. Whereas art had always saved her before, she found now that she could no longer paint. She attempted suicide again and checked herself into a hospital.

Fortunately, Kusama worked with a doctor who was interested in the benefits of **art therapy.** She found that thanks to the structure and safety of the institution, she could create again.

This would be a good place to stop for a happy ending, but to do so would be simplifying the reality of things. Kusama still lives in a mental health institution. When she attends her exhibitions, a psychiatrist travels with her. She is not cured but instead says that she is "managing madness."[17]

To some extent, then, Kusama has perhaps allowed her mental illness to limit or control her life. But you could also look at it another way: she has created a controlled environment in which she can do the one thing that she always wanted to do, which is create her art. Kusama has literally created her own worlds, with huge installations and detailed large-scale paintings, a universe in which she is empowered, in which the work emerges exactly as it is supposed to be, and in which trauma is limited because exposure to her fears is carefully controlled. Art has ultimately made Kusama's life not just bearable, but beautiful.

Institutional Racism & Trauma

In the same way that war is a type of trauma that can be passed down generationally, living in a society upheld by the structures of institutional racism is also a form of trauma. Beyond tackling the complex subject of racial trauma from a political or historical perspective, many contemporary artists are addressing the psychological damage that stems from traumatic racism on a deeply personal level—efforts that have done much to destigmatize discussions of mental health.

For example, in her performance art project *The Body Remembers* Black British artist Heather Agyepong explores how trauma lives in the body, particularly for Black British women across different generations, and the power of healing through therapeutic movement.[1] Agyepong says of dealing with the subject of mental health in her work: "There is a general taboo around the subject. I wanted to contribute to the conversation as I don't want the future generation having any blocks to these conversations and seeking help."[2]

Another example is painter Malik Roberts series *Blk and Blue,* in which he uses a monochromatic blue palette to showcase how mental health is a a universal issue, as well as cultural signifiers that suggest it's a problem that must be addressed specifically in Black communities. His paintings explore "the ways PTSD, anxiety, depression, and bipolar disorder manifest in communities afflicted by poverty, racism, broken windows policing, and violence."[3]

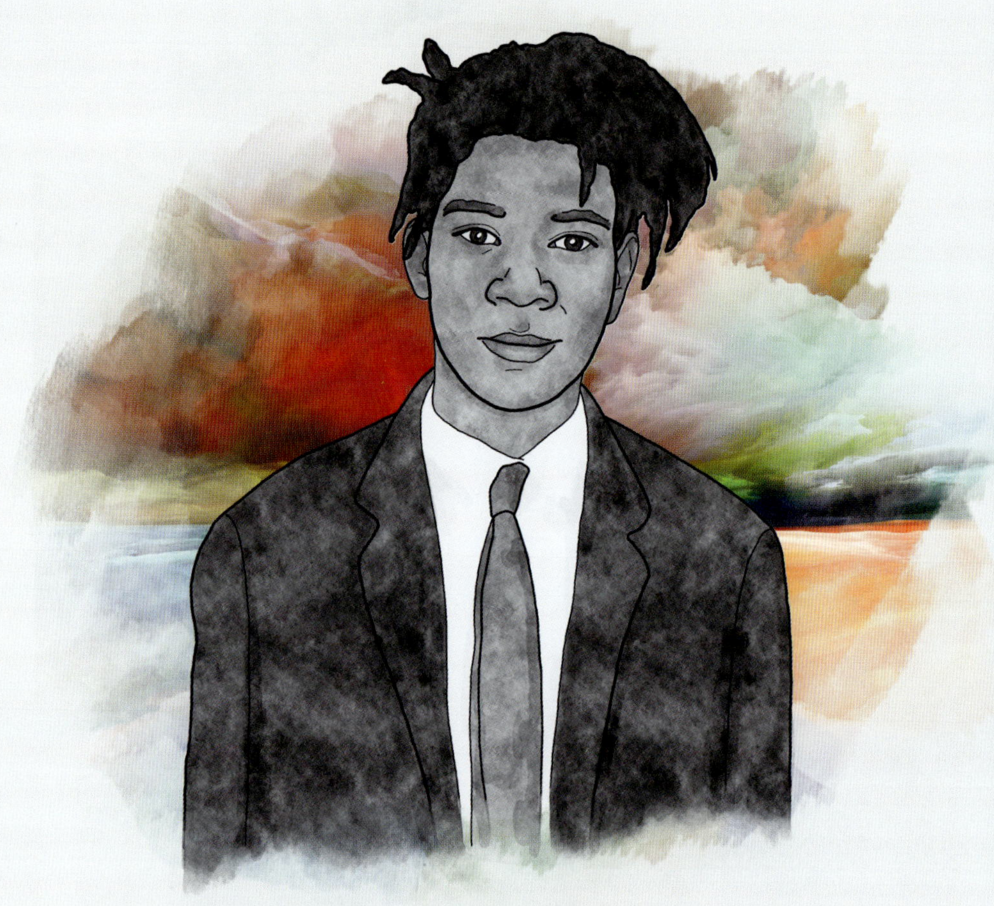

Jean-Michel Basquiat

(December 22, 1960–August 12, 1988)

I had some money; I made the best paintings ever. I was completely reclusive, worked a lot, took a lot of drugs. I was awful to people.

—JEAN-MICHEL BASQUIAT[1]

Jean-Michel Basquiat is a bit of an enigma. On one hand, we have access to a lot of information about him due in part to the fact that he lived relatively recently and was famous. And yet, because his persona was so well known, it's difficult to separate the myth from the man. He himself once said, upon hearing Elton John's *Candle in the Wind* (which is about Marilyn Monroe), "That's me. I'm not a real person. I'm a legend."[2]

Because of this, the relationship between Basquiat's art and mental health is difficult to parse, complicated further by the fact that he died very young, at the age of twenty-seven from a drug overdose. However, it's apparent that his drug use was an attempt to **self-medicate**—a common approach to dealing with undiagnosed mental illness and trauma.

Basquiat began using drugs at least as early as age fifteen. Even if he had sought mental health treatment, it would be a challenge for a professional to parse out which symptoms might be due to a disorder, and which might be attributed to the effects of drugs on his developing brain. **Dual diagnosis** (the term for when a person has both a substance abuse issue and another mental health issue) requires specific treatment to separate out and treat both problems.[3] As you figure out what symptoms are related to which issue, you may treat the substance abuse first, the mood disorder first, or both concurrently. This "chicken or the egg" situation often makes treatment complicated. We do know that he had a history of trauma, which no doubt influenced his mental health and his art.

The first trauma in Basquiat's life, and the most vivid memory he recalls having, was an accident that happened when he was around seven years old.[4] He was hit by a car, had to have his spleen removed, and spent at least a month in bed recuperating.[5] In examining other artists, such as Yayoi Kusama or Frida Kahlo, we have seen how repetition can emerge as a theme in their art as a way to process trauma, and images of cars and ambulances would recur in Basquiat's work throughout his life. We can draw a direct comparison here to Kahlo's traumatic bus accident, and the many self-portraits she painted of herself recovering in bed. Interestingly, Basquiat spent his time healing immersed in a book that would also become relevant to his later art. His mother, Mathilde, an art lover who often took Basquiat to museums, gave him a copy of *Gray's Anatomy*, which he loved to flip through and marvel at the anatomical sketches.[6] This is another parallel with Kahlo, who contemplated becoming a medical illustrator and often incorporated anatomical renderings in her work. It's no wonder that two artists who were traumatically injured at a young age would display a preoccupation with the body.

A passion for art was not the only legacy Basquiat's mother left him. Mathilde had mental health issues, and her time in and out of institutions led to more trauma for the young artist. He described her as having recurrent depression and that she was sometimes violent. Basquiat's father, Gerard, confirms that Matilde assaulted him, once trying to stab him with a knife.[7] In addition to the numerous stories Basquiat recounted about her violence toward his father, he recalled that when he was in kindergarten and put his underwear on backward, she beat him "for the longest time."[8]

This was not the only family issue. Basquiat's father, Gerard, was an immigrant from Haiti. His family was well off but encountered political issues that landed both of Jean-Michel's grandparents in jail.[9] Gerard's brother (Jean-Michel's uncle) was murdered.[10] The trauma of imprisonment, death, and loss echoed through the family. As we've seen with other artists, such as Mark Rothko, intergenerational trauma can be a contributing factor to mental health issues.[11]

Basquiat's childhood home was not a happy one. Gerard and Mathilde obviously had a troubled relationship and eventually divorced. The children lived with their dad; however, Jean-Michel struggled to get along with his father. Neighbors described Gerard as strict, self-absorbed, and lacking the ability to understand his son. "Strict" might be a gross understatement—Jean-Michel reported Gerard to the police for stabbing him and beating his sisters.[12] While his father and at least one of his sisters denied these claims, neighbors, friends, and teachers have corroborated them, citing that Jean-Michel once came to school walking with a cane after one of the assaults.[13] Basquiat had additional trauma outside the home. He told friends that his first sexual experience was oral rape by an older adult man.[14] He had always had problems at school, and they unsurprisingly began to get worse after this experience. People in his life noticed a shift in him; the owner of a local flower shop where Basquiat spent time recalls, "He went from a sweet, trusting boy to someone who was very, very guarded and moody, bordering on hostile."[15] It is understandable that Basquiat left home for good at seventeen.

Basquiat told a school friend that while homeless he sometimes did sex work for money, and that he possibly contracted syphilis from one of these interactions. Apparently, he said this while laughing, seemingly disconnected from the experience.[16] Children who experience early sexual trauma may become ongoing victims of similar trauma, and at times they turn to sex work because it gives them a sense of control over the abuse. Oftentimes these experiences only further traumatize the victim of abuse. Due to cultural stigma, it would have been challenging for Basquiat to report, discuss, and heal from this type of trauma. Many sexual-abuse victims don't speak up right away for a variety of reasons; boys, in particular, are less likely to report abuse because of our society's masculine gender norms that exacerbate the shame. Black boys in particular are an underserved population when it comes to getting help for sexual abuse. Nikitta A. Foston, writing for *Ebony,* explains:

> Because African-American boys are in an environment that applauds "macho-ism," they feel powerless when they are violated and they feel as though they have failed themselves by allowing something like this to happen. So many young men who haven't been exposed to anything other than abuse think it is simply a part of life.[17]

Considering all this abuse and trauma, it is no wonder Basquiat struggled with his mental health. The artist was frequently described as mercurial or moody. One critic said his personality was "both charming and disdainful."[18] Ex-girlfriend Valda Grinfelds said, "He was a brilliant painter, a horrible egotist, he was a total selfish brat, he was a kind, gentle, pained spirit, he was a hurt little boy, an arrogant old man, and everything in between."[19] Vrej Baghoomian, his final agent, said that Basquiat was always in emotional torment.[20] These tensions in his personality perhaps explain why, though Basquiat had passionate relationships with friends, he also has a history of falling out with them. **Early-childhood attachment issues** due to his troubled home also likely contributed to his pattern of troubled adult relationships.

Basquiat's most public friendship "breakup" was with Andy Warhol. He had always wanted to know Warhol. Once, while still an unknown street artist, he approached Warhol and sold him some of his art, but he didn't make much of an impression on the celebrity artist at the time. Later, Basquiat was introduced to Warhol at a restaurant and impressed the older man when he abruptly left and returned an hour later with a painted portrait of the two of them together. They became good friends for a time and worked on a collaborative art series, though it was not well received.[21] The press essentially painted Basquiat to be Warhol's lapdog.[22] As a result, Basquiat may have begun to believe that Warhol was taking advantage of him. Friends report that he was becoming increasingly paranoid at this time, possibly due to drug use. However, his worries were not entirely unwarranted, since many people did try to take advantage of his rising star. In any case, Basquiat and Warhol stopped speaking. Before the rift could be remedied, Warhol died, and Basquiat was inconsolable.[23]

Jay Shriver, one of Andy Warhol's painting assistants, believed that Basquiat specifically sought out friendship with Warhol because he needed validation from someone of his stature in the art world to "overcome his insecurities as an artist."[24] We often spend our lives trying to cope with and repair early-childhood wounds, and this relationship may have been a form of repetition compulsion. A school friend noted that Basquiat "craved parental approval."[25] In fact, despite the childhood abuse, Basquiat stayed in touch with both of his parents and frequently seemed to attempt to get their positive attention. Gallerist and art dealer Mary Boone believed that Basquiat cared too much about what others thought about him, and therefore had trouble holding his center in the midst of all of the celebrity and chaos that became his life.[26]

Basquiat was prolific in his short lifetime. He was known to paint quickly, even feverishly, and, as his fame grew, he was forced to increase that speed.[27] Phoebe Hoban elaborates on some of the power dynamics at play between Basquiat and his dealers:

> The lonely, alienated, and disenfranchised artist whose constant need to produce—out of his own untrammeled creativity, deep-seated desire for approval,

> and insatiable demand for the cash that would buy him drugs—became their ready source of profit.[28]

As Basquiat churned out paintings for the consumption and profit of the larger art world, critics wondered if the fast pace would lead to burnout. Basquiat idolized creatives such as Jimi Hendrix and Charlie Parker, who "lived fast and died young" but left the world a wealth of inspired work in their wake.[28]

In addition to the commodification of his art, Basquiat himself was treated as a sort of mascot for the carnivorous art industry, and he felt the pain of this acutely. Yes, he was celebrated, but in many ways his work was also fetishized, even by his detractors. Art critic Robert Hughes said that the art world accepted him only because they yearned to buy work from an "urban noble savage."[29] Even admirers of Basquiat's art often described it in overly simplistic terms. In one awkward exchange, an interviewer asks about his work being "primitive," and Basquiat responds, "Like a primate? Do you mean like an ape?" The white interviewer stumbles over a response. In another interview, Basquiat tells the camera that people see him as a "wild monkey man," and explicitly calls out the art world as racist.[30] Many biographies and documentaries note the tragic irony that even when he was earning thousands of dollars per painting and wearing Armani suits, as a Black man he still had trouble getting a taxi in 1980s Manhattan.[31]

Basquiat incorporated the theme of trauma related to identity, racism, and exploitation into his work. For example, in 1983 he painted *The Death of Michael Stewart* in response to the death of his friend. Michael Stewart was a young Black graffiti artist who was beaten to death by six white New York policemen, all of whom were later acquitted.[32] Basquiat unsurprisingly identified with Stewart and was tortured by the news.[33] He had been addressing police violence in his work for several years; *Irony of a Negro Policeman*, painted in 1981, questions how a Black man could participate in a system so oppressive to his own people. We have become increasingly aware in recent years of the trauma inflicted on Black communities by police brutality specifically, and systemic racism on a larger scale, and it is important to take into account this trauma understanding Basquiat's personal struggle.

The more money Basquiat made, the more drugs he consumed. By 1985, "he had used so much cocaine he'd perforated his septum," though he would find ways to sober up from time to time.[34] Reportedly, his friendship with Warhol helped him reduce his intake, with the older man trying to convince him to stay clean.[35] One of the few documented instances of Basquiat specifically referring to his own mental health was when he confided to Warhol, who wrote in his journal, "Jean-Michel came by and said he was depressed and was going to kill himself[,] and I laughed and said it was just because he hadn't slept for four days."[36] Warhol's death not only left Basquiat free-floating in his own grief but also left him floundering without the paternalistic oversight that reigned in his drug use.[37] Although he had once been a prolific painter, the late stages of his drug addiction kept him from finishing commissions.[38] Even as the drugs were eroding his ability to work, Basquiat believed that he couldn't create without them.[39]

That said, Basquiat claimed in those last months that he had his drug use under control, though friends were skeptical. Basquiat seemed to have a strong desire to get sober. He attempted rehab at one point, but, according to ex-girlfriend Jennifer Goode, he simply couldn't abide "all those white doctors and psychiatrists, telling him what to do," and became instead determined to get off the drugs on his own.[40] He did not succeed, dying less than two years after Warhol.

Extraordinarily prolific and dedicated to his work, Basquiat seemed to understand that art making was the best way of coping with his trauma, but sadly he found drug use as a coping mechanism as well.

Gender Identity and Dysphoria

Gender dysphoria describes a type of distress experienced when there is a mismatch between one's biological sex and their gender identity. You may have heard "born in the wrong body" as a way to describe the gender dysphoria felt by some transgender people. Gender identity can be even more complex and nuanced, with societal expectations of masculinity and femininity leaving many feeling uneasy in their own bodies due to the restrictive nature of our culture's ideas around gender presentation. As such, terms such as "gender fluidity" and "non-binary" have entered the lexicon to help people better describe their personal experience of gender beyond the binary.

Expressing thoughts and feelings about gender through art can be a safe and productive way to explore one's identity, which is especially important since gender dysphoria is linked to depression and other mood disorders.[1] Claude Cahun, a pioneering French queer creative who lived during the first half of the twentieth century, is one example. Through strikingly modern genderbending and performative self-portraits, Cahun opens the door for possible identities that were not available to them in society at the time. As art historian Tirza True Latimer describes: "They were in the mode of investigation, who you could be, how you could be, projecting yourself into another skin, another universe . . . The photographs, the acting out, were a way of being free."[2]

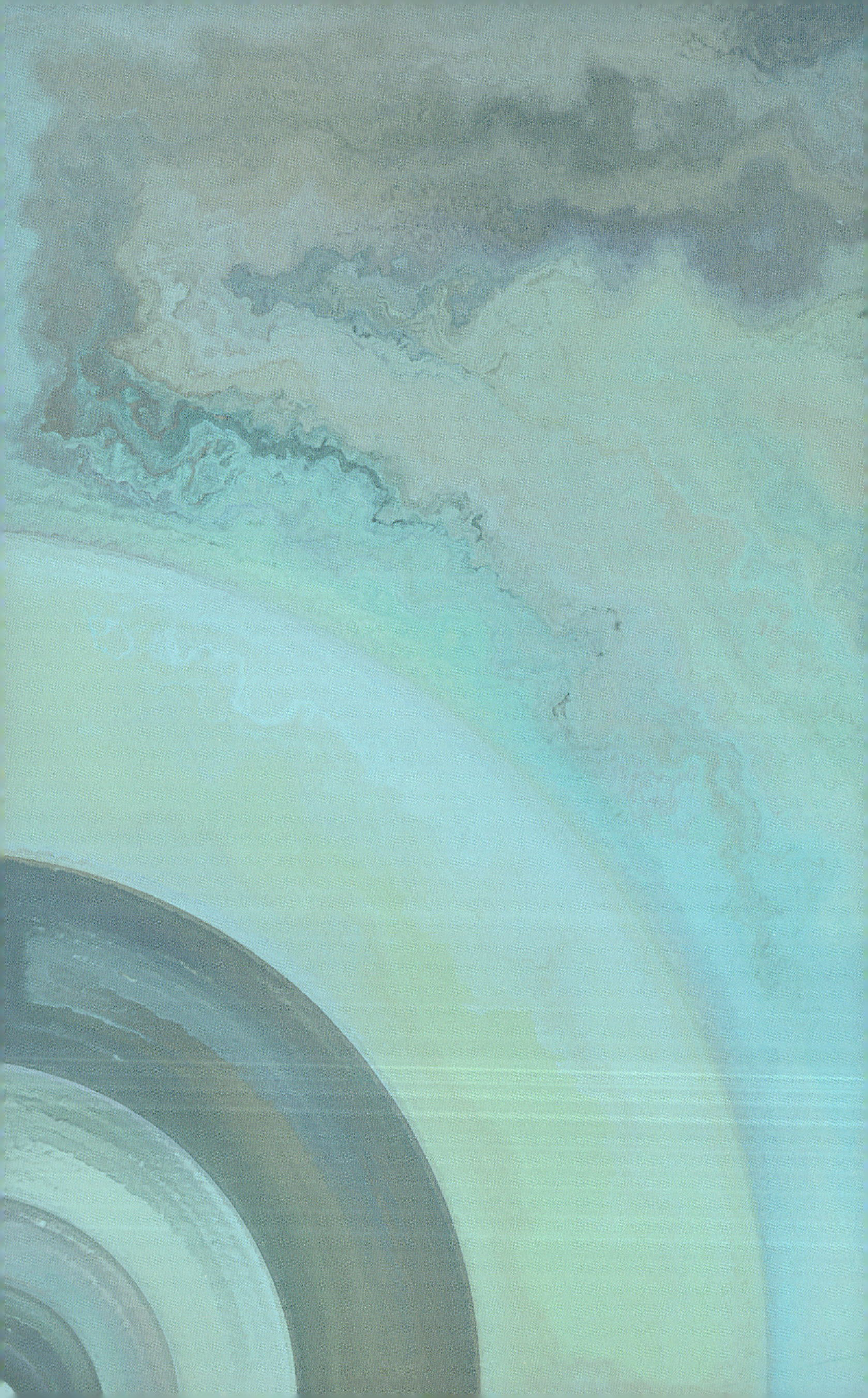

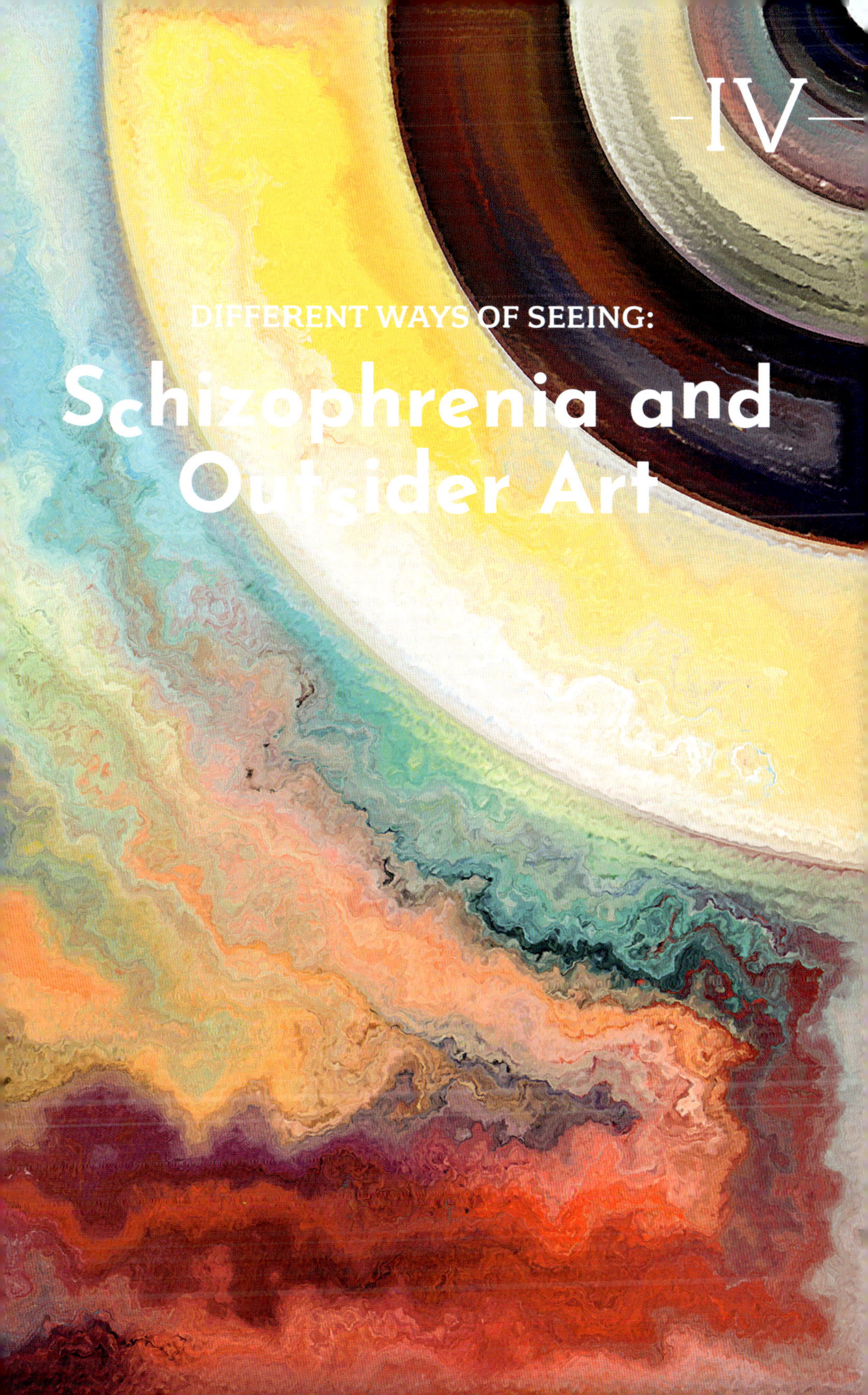
-IV-
DIFFERENT WAYS OF SEEING:
Schizophrenia and
Outsider Art

Let's turn to the diagnosis of schizophrenia or a disorder on the schizophrenia spectrum. A strikingly large percentage of so-called outsider artists have this diagnosis. Schizophrenia is one of the most feared and stigmatized mental health issues to this day; when people think of someone "going crazy," they picture the worst symptoms of schizophrenia—hallucinations, delusions, and even violence. While there can be extreme symptoms, and it is a challenging condition to treat, people with schizophrenia can also live long, fulfilling, and creative lives.

WHAT IS SCHIZOPHRENIA?

Schizophrenia is a chronic, long-term mental health condition in which the individual has trouble distinguishing among thought, emotion, and behavior. This results in a variety of different symptoms, but it is essentially a breakdown in the ability to distinguish reality from imagination, delusion, or hallucination. It's as though there's a blurring or disconnect between what's occurring in the world and what's happening in the brain.

There are three categories of schizophrenia symptoms: psychosis, cognitive symptoms, and negative symptoms. People most often associate schizophrenia with **psychotic symptoms**, specifically auditory and visual hallucinations. Psychotic symptoms also include delusions, which are fixed beliefs that are at odds with objective reality. Paranoia is a common example—the belief that someone is "out to get you." Disordered thinking and unusual speech patterns are also symptoms of psychosis. These are sometimes called "positive symptoms," which doesn't mean they are good, but instead that they are symptoms not normally present for the average person.

Cognitive symptoms in schizophrenia are similar to those in other mental health disorders and include difficulty focusing, concentrating, and making decisions, as well as problems with memory. People with schizophrenia may find it hard to learn new things, and they have difficulty using or accepting information they are given. These are sometimes also called disorganized symptoms.

Finally, there are **negative symptoms**, which refers to the absence of something. For example, people with schizophrenia may lack interest in activities, have trouble finding motivation, or be devoid of emotional expression. They may be unable to plan, begin, or continue activities, and they may have a flat affect, with both a monotone voice and a neutral facial expression. Some people with severe symptoms may even stop speaking altogether.

Although subtle signs of the illness may emerge in childhood and teen years, people usually get diagnosed with schizophrenia in their twenties or thirties, with men tending to present symptoms slightly earlier than women. Often a person receives the diagnosis after their first major experience with symptoms of psychosis, though psychosis itself is not always indicative of schizophrenia. Bipolar depression can manifest with psychotic symptoms in extreme manic phases, and drug use can cause psychotic symptoms, including paranoia. So, it's not always easy to make a diagnosis of schizophrenia, and someone's presenting symptoms may not always fit the exact label. But, generally speaking, people with schizophrenia will have hallucinations, disordered thinking, and difficulty relating thoughts, feelings, and behavior in a typical way.

"OUTSIDER ART": REAL OR MYTH?

Probably no art so caters to the public's hatred of the establishment as outsider art. The work of the uneducated, the insane, the criminal and the underprivileged, outsider art preserves a myth of esthetic purity for a culture tired of its experts. The outsider artist has not suffered the deforming influence of art school, and his art requires no esoteric explanation from critics. Motivated merely by the joy of making art, the outsider is totally unaware, or so the story goes, of the history of art or of the marketplace.

–WENDY STEINER, *NEW YORK TIMES*[1]

"Outsider art" is a problematic term, and yet, it is one that's been historically widely accepted, so it's important that we dissect it before we further explore artists who may (or may not) fall into this category. In brief, the term refers to art created outside the traditional, formally and socially sanctioned art world. If many contemporary artists take a path that includes earning an MFA, interning or apprenticing with higher-ups in the art world, achieving gallery representation with an eye on sales and exhibitions, etc., then outsider art is the opposite: **self-taught artists working outside those boundaries without connection to or perhaps even any knowledge of the traditionally accepted Western societal realm or industry termed "the art market."** That's the basics. However, when we delve deeper into who exactly gets labeled an "outsider artist," it becomes clear why the term is controversial, and how it directly links with societal perceptions of mental illness and the stigmatization of various groups.

An idea essentially coined by French artist Jean Dubuffet in the 1940s, who called it "art brut," which translates to "raw art," this style of work was renamed "outsider art" in the 1970s by art critic Roger Cardinal.[2] Dubuffet was captivated with art made by people in psychiatric institutions, and was specifically inspired by the writings of German psychiatrist and art historian Hans Prinzhorn, which documented a wide array of asylum art. Dubuffet was also fascinated with artwork by prisoners, mediums or clairvoyants, children, the elderly, and the uneducated.[3] Subsequently, those who champion so-called outsider art have continued to focus on art created in institutional settings (by psychiatric patients as well as incarcerated people), along with art created by people with learning disabilities or mental health challenges, those experiencing homelessness, and other marginalized groups.

We can immediately see the problems with this label from the broad spectrum of artists included under its umbrella. While it's certainly wonderful to acknowledge these artists in their own right, the history of the art world's engagement with outsider art has been marked by a sort of patronizing privilege. In the same way that we would never say today that Christopher Columbus "discovered" America, it's also problematic to say that someone from the art world (such as a critic, dealer, or curator) has "discovered" an outsider artist. There is also an issue with insisting that outsider art is somehow "pure" or "untouched," as if all the diverse artists who would supposedly fit into this category have no understanding of the world around them, and that their work is not just as contextual to specific cultural and social moments as the work of artists accepted by the establishment.

In an effort to correct the offensive terminology, art such as this has more recently been called **"self-taught" or "visionary" art**. In the 1990s, Baltimore opened the American Visionary Art Museum, a place for "visionary and outsider art," recognized by Congress as art "produced by self-taught individuals who are driven by their own internal impulses to create."[4] The language here, and what originally drew Dubuffet and Cardinal to this work, suggests there is something special about **art created purely to fulfill the desire to self-express**, as opposed to work that caters to the whims of the art world and is made in order to make a living. That point could perhaps be argued, but in the years since the movement has gained popularity, so-called outsider art often ends up just as mediated by the market as mainstream art, due to the influence of dealers, buyers, and an interested public.[5] The biannual Outsider Art Fair, held in New York and Paris and accompanied each year by a dedicated Christie's sale, is one example of the diminishing difference in markets (the owner of the fair, Andrew Edlin, estimates the outsider art market generates as much as between $40 million and $50 million each year[6]).

We could delve more deeply into the topic of outsider art, since there is extensive critical research dissecting the term and its history; however, most of that scholarship is outside the scope of this book. What we can't neglect is the direct relationship between mental health stigmatization and the appellation of outsider art. As we've seen in the previous chapters, people can live, work, and create despite devastating mental illness, so simply having a mental illness does not automatically qualify one as an outsider artist, however fraught the term.

Historically, a white male could exhibit signs of mental illness—and even spend time in an asylum—and still be an accepted, even canonical artist (Vincent van Gogh being the obvious example). Women and people of color less so, often achieving acceptance only if somehow associated with notable white men. For many, recognition came later, thanks to revisionist art-historical studies with a focus on gender and race. As Wendy Steiner puts it:

> There is not a single criterion of "outsiderness" that cannot be found in "inside" artists. Van Gogh was mad. Joseph Cornell was self-taught. Caravaggio was a criminal. El Greco was a visionary. Socially deviant high artists like Jean-Michel Basquiat are a dime a dozen. Chagall's paintings are as full of fanciful folk elements as any outsider artist's work, and everyone from Duchamp to Rauschenberg has made art out of scraps and refuse.[7]

Oftentimes, the artists who managed to "make it" are those who have a combination of privilege and access that make it easier to live with their symptoms and achieve acceptance as an "insider." Richard Dadd was white, male, and affluent, so despite ending up in a psychiatric hospital for patricide, he was never considered an "outsider artist."

Moreover, mental health is incredibly nuanced, and with so much gray area, the broad term of outsider art does a disservice to the individual. How do we categorize Yayoi Kusama, for example, in the context of outsider art? In many ways she was an outsider in the New York art world, being both a woman and Japanese, but she did manage to navigate that world to great success. Yet, she has lived and created in a psychiatric institution for decades. Had she not managed to make a name for herself first, had someone else happened to notice her work at the asylum and promote it, would she then be considered an "outsider artist"? Then there is Diane Arbus, who was born into privilege but felt like an outsider and arguably tried to make herself one by photographing people in the fringes of society. Yet, she still always kept one foot in the world of her birth, continuing to photograph friends, celebrities, and the wealthy at the same time.[8] Can you cross from "insider" to "outsider" by choice?

It's a tricky thing to define all of this. **One suggestion is to banish the binary and instead place artists on a spectrum from "outsider" to "mainstream,"** a solution that at least recognizes that it's a blurry distinction influenced by a person's education, psychology, status in society, and many other factors.[9] How to actually define the points along that spectrum is also a murky endeavor, but it's better than the black-and-white notion of being either "in" or "out." These issues are worth keeping in mind as we explore the artists in this section, because their relative access to services and support may have played a key role not only in the treatment of their mental health challenges, but in how their artistic lives unfolded as well.

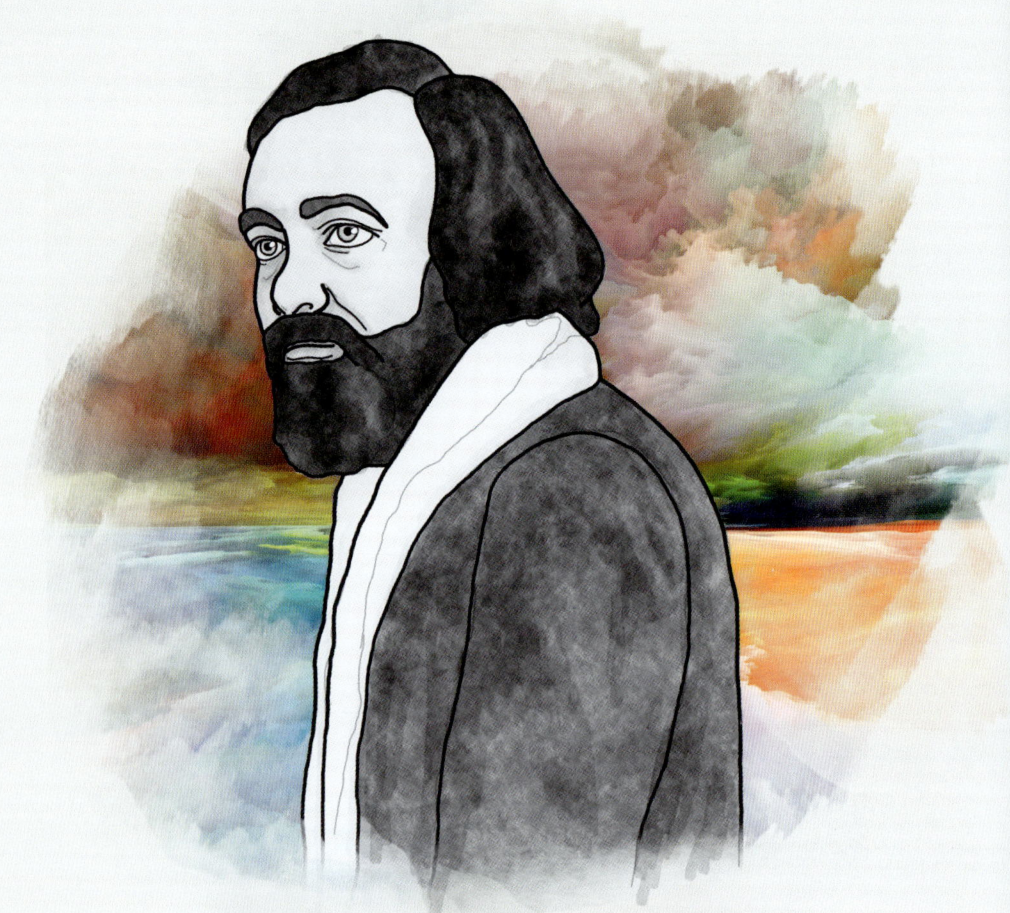

Richard Dadd

(August 1, 1817–January 7, 1886)

I had such ideas that, had I spoken of them openly, I must, if answered in the world's fashion, have been told I was unreasonable. I concealed, of course, these secret admonitions. I knew not whence they came, although I could not question their propriety, nor could I separate myself from what appeared my fate.

—RICHARD DADD[1]

In his midtwenties, Richard Dadd took a trip that precipitated a lifetime of mental illness and simultaneously set the tone for most of what he would paint in the decades to come.[2] Dadd had shown budding promise as an artist and began studying at London's Royal Academy of Arts.[3] He had some success with his first paintings, which were of fairies. At twenty-six, he was commissioned by Sir Thomas Phillips to take a long trip together, for the artist to draw what he saw during the trek.[4] During the ten-month expedition, Dadd grew increasingly angry with others, began to have delusions, and threatened to murder the pope.[5] After visiting Syria, Dadd wrote a letter to a friend in which he said his imagination was "so full of vagaries" that he doubted his own sanity.[6] Their travels proceeded to Egypt, after which Dadd wrote that he experienced nearly a week of nervous depression, the reason for which he couldn't understand.

When Dadd returned home to England, the delusions overtook him. His behavior changed, he adopted an odd diet of only ale and eggs, and people had difficulty understanding him when he talked.[7] A doctor diagnosed Dadd with "an aberration of the intellect" and recommended psychiatric care, but his father declined to get him professional help. That was a mistake for Richard, but even more so for his father—during a walk in the park, Richard murdered him by stabbing him in the chest and slitting his throat.[8] Dadd later said he believed that his father had been possessed by the devil, and that he was acting under the instructions of the god of Osiris when he committed the crime.[9] Richard immediately fled to Dover and then to France, but en route from Calais to Paris he again fell victim to a delusion, attacked a stranger with a razor, and was subsequently arrested.[10] Later, he confessed that he had fled with the intention of finding and murdering Ferdinand I, the emperor of Austria.[11] Dadd was diagnosed with "homicidal monomania" due to emotional trauma. With his hallucinations and delusions, his modern-day diagnosis would likely be schizophrenia with delusions of religiosity.[12] However, the term "schizophrenia" wasn't developed until after Dadd's death, first used by Eugene Bleuler in 1908.[13] Whereas Leonora Carrington had a nonviolent breakdown but recovered and didn't have further issues, Dadd continued to have delusions for the rest of his life.

Dadd spent the next four decades of his life in the psychiatric prisons of England, first at the Bedlam Hospital and later, as psychiatrist Allan Beveridge describes, at a "new state-of-the-art asylum built at Broadmoor near Reading in Berkshire especially for the criminally insane following the introduction of new legislation in the Criminal Lunatics Asylum Act of 1860."[14] His mental health continued to decline, his delusions only worsening with age.[15] Throughout his time in the asylum, Dadd would occasionally become violent and would "binge eat until he vomited, and otherwise behave eccentrically, believing that he was possessed of special powers."[16]

As explored in depth in the book *Masters of Bedlam: The Transformation of the Mad-Doctoring Trade*, it was an intriguing time in the history of mental health treatment. "Only after 1800 did systematic provision begin to be made for segregating the insane into specialized institutions."[17] While certainly many terrible things took place in these asylums, there were also, for the first time, sincere attempts to provide therapy to the institutionalized, and art was one of those forms of therapy (as were music lessons, gymnastics, language classes, and allowing patients to keep animals as pets).[18] In Dadd's case, he was given his own art studio and allowed to paint, so he devoted most of his time to making art.[19] He did not paint in his first year, which was "one of great agitation."[20] But then, he began to paint prolifically, an activity that seemed to bring him a sense of calm.[21]

Dadd spent nine years adding paint to his masterpiece *The Fairy Feller's Master-Stroke*, so thickly applied onto the canvas that it became three-dimensional and the strange figures sprang to life.[22] Because of this, you can really grasp the detail of this piece only if you see it in person, and even then it's hard to capture all of the nuance. To call

Dadd detail-oriented would be an understatement; one author describes him as "a painter of microscopic refinement."[23] In completing this piece, he would work on one tiny section at a time, drawing a detailed sketch, then painstakingly applying paint to that area. He would go over and over the spot, layering on paint, which altered the perspective, adding to the magical quality of the fairyland.[24] The artwork is fantastical, but it is also haunting. For one thing, it depicts a patriarch wearing a triple crown, which seems to be a reference to the pope. It also includes an apothecary that is a portrait of the artist's father. Neither of these characters seems particularly sinister if you don't know the backstory, but since Dadd threatened to kill the pope and did actually murder his father, it lends intensity to the work. Was the artist trying to process his homicidal delusions, or even perhaps his guilt, through his art? We'll never know exactly, though the main character, who holds an ax that he never finished painting, bears some physical similarity to Dadd himself.[25]

In Dadd's lifetime there were no antipsychotic medications and thus little chance that he would be rehabilitated to the point he could safely exist in society. Even the most-progressive hospitals, such as the asylum where he stayed, used dubious treatments such as cold baths to try to resolve serious mental illness.[26] However, Dadd is an example of someone who was able to keep contributing to the world through art, even while imprisoned. Seemingly unsure whether people would understand this elaborate work that he took years to complete, Dadd later wrote a poem about *Fairy Feller*, trying to explain in words what the imagery is all about. In addition to the pope and the apothecary, there are hundreds of other characters in the painting. One writer describes them as delusions that visited Dadd: "His visitants were not great men, not sages, heroes, or martyrs; but goggle-eyed gnomes, and malicious fays and tormenting Pucks, and pot-bellied, spindle shanked brownies."[27] It's a long poem that reads like what it is—the ramblings of someone with lifelong schizophrenic delusions.

Nevertheless, people were inspired by *Fairy Feller* and continued to be for years. Most famously, Freddie Mercury of Queen wrote a song about it, with lyrics straight from Dadd's poem.[28] Octavio Paz and Neil Gaiman are two well-known writers who have cited the piece's influence.[29] But perhaps the most interesting work that describes this painting is a book by Lesley Krueger called *Mad Richard*, which is a strange work of historical fiction in which Charlotte Bronte's life is intertwined with Dadd's. In this work, real characters merge with fiction, which seems poignant since the schizophrenic mind often has trouble distinguishing between what is real and what is imagined.

While *Fairy Feller* became the most famous, there are several other paintings that similarly provide insight into the artist's mind. For example, consider *The Flight Out of Egypt*. Remember that the artist's first serious break with reality happened during his travels, particularly in and around Egypt. It's little wonder, then, that his expression of that experience is the chaos of another completely filled canvas. There seems to be no particular focus to this work. In fact, Dadd didn't even give it a name.[30] It's as though he never came to terms with this initial break in his mind. A preoccupation with his own delusions shows up even more clearly in paintings that aren't derived from his memory. For example, Dadd did a series of pictures in the 1950s called "The Passions," featuring such titles as *Hatred* and *Agony*, prompting one writer to say, "If in his landscapes, portraits and Shakespearean fantasies he was partly remembering a world others could recognise, in these he has turned inwards."[31]

One hallmark of art made by those with schizophrenia is the repetition of themes,[32] and Dadd repeatedly painted symbols from his own hallucinations that began in Egypt. Indeed, although the amount of time that Dadd actually spent in Egypt was brief, the experience of his delusions there became a nearly obsessive focus of his mind and art for the rest of his life, as seen in *The Flight Out of Egypt*.[33] Another piece in which we see themes and symbols from Egypt is *Halt in the Desert*. He painted this work in 1845, marking the beginning of his art making in the asylum.[34] It depicts an evening the artist camped along the Dead Sea, which we know from his writings was a fraught time in that already-challenging journey. At first glance, this deceptively peaceful scene in the desert looks calm and inviting, thanks to the soft light of the moon and fire that give it an almost cozy glow. But Dadd was already experiencing hallucinations during this trip. Some suggest that the reason *Halt in the Desert* looks so calm is because the artist longed for a more peaceful state of mind, and that the work was "calculated to impress on an excited brain, calming its horror and lulling its rage to sleep."[35] This draws parallels with the calm scenes from nature in Georgia O'Keeffe's work, the stillness of a remembered landscape perhaps easing the artists' anxieties.

Finally, there is one more Richard Dadd painting that serves as a key to unlock the story of his mental illness: the portrait of *Sir Alexander*

Morison, 1779—1866, Alienist (alienist is a historical term for a psychologist or psychiatrist). Dadd met Sir Alexander Morison, the man depicted in the painting, in a psychiatric prison, and perhaps Dadd's own mental distress at his situation accounts for the anguish that permeates the image.[36] How distressed Sir Alexander Morison appears as well, because he was going through a terrible time when he commissioned the painting. Morison had held high hopes for his career, and retroactive accolades have been given to his contributions to psychological treatments. However, when alive he struggled considerably, both to gain respect and to make money. During his lifetime, he was regularly compared to his peer, another psychiatrist and medical lecturer named John Conolly, and never too favorably.[37]

In the painting, Morison is shown standing in front of his family estate in Edinburgh. Of course, since Dadd was locked up for most of his life, he certainly never saw the man there. He painted that part of the image on the basis of a sketch that Morison's own daughter had drawn.[38] One of Morison's descendants included a copy of the image in a book about the family, saying that it really isn't the best likeness of the man but that he liked how the background was depicted. Dadd added fisherwomen in the background, likely painted from photos by David Octavius Hill and Robert Adamson, who were "pioneering Scottish photographers."[39] So, even though Dadd was painting someone he knew very well, the image looks a little bit "off" because so much of the composition is drawn from images by other people, and of things that Dadd never saw in person. Again, there is an eeriness from the merging of reality and the imagined emanating from this work that reflects the multiple dimensions of the schizophrenic mind.

Richard Dadd lived out the rest of his life at the Broadmoor asylum. He contracted and died of tuberculosis there at the age of sixty-eight and was buried on the grounds.[40] Many mental health issues, including schizophrenia, are genetic, and this seems to be the case for Dadd. He was one of seven children, four of whom "would eventually die insane."[41]

Dadd's work was little recognized in his lifetime, excepting some attention to *Fairy Feller*.[42] In this way, he could be considered an outsider artist. He created his art in an asylum and was "discovered" later in life. He's not labeled as such, though, and his overwhelming privilege as a white male born into an educated, affluent family is more than likely the reason.[43] It was in the 1960s when his work began to get more-widespread attention, particularly from the antipsychiatry movement headed up by R. D. Laing. The movement questioned the practices of asylums (such as electroshock therapy treatments), argued against many mental health diagnoses (such as homosexuality, which was still considered a mental illness at the time), and argued for the rights of the mentally ill.[44] Dadd became a bit of a hero to this group, since "his artistic accomplishments in this environment were seen as a triumph over adversity" by those who were in favor of the elimination of the Victorian-era asylum.[45] That said, at least one writer has argued that the environment of the asylum actually aided Dadd's artistic pursuits, saying "Dadd's work testifies to the care and support of his doctors in the shelter of the asylum, where he was freed from having to satisfy the demands of artistic fashion."[46] In other words, it's possible his status as an institutionalized outsider is what made room for his creativity.

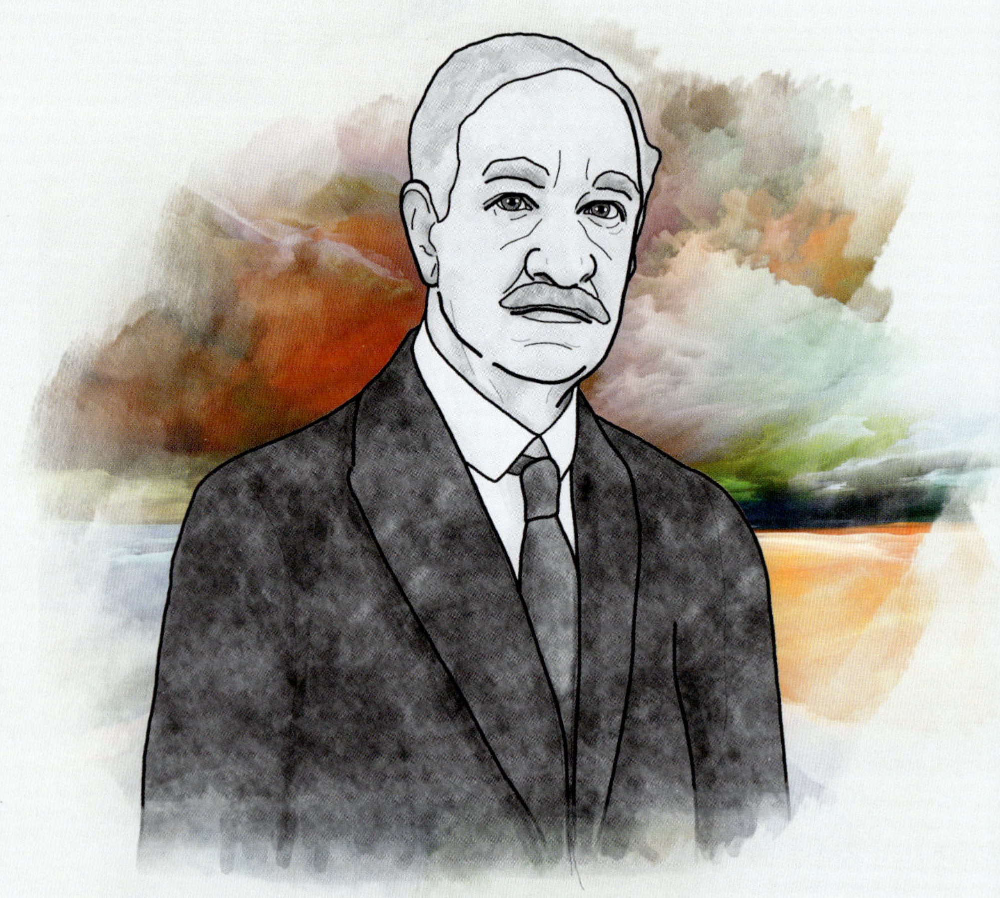

Louis Wain

(August 5, 1860–July 4, 1939)

I seemed to live hundreds of years, and to see thousands of mental pictures of extraordinary complexity. . . . But above all, I was haunted; in the streets, at home, by day and night, by a vast globe, which seemed to have endless surface, and I seemed to see myself climbing over and over it, until, from sheer fright I came to myself, and the vision went.

–LOUIS WAIN[1]

As we move on to the next artist, keep in mind two important things about schizophrenia. First, it almost always manifests when someone is in their twenties and thirties, rarely earlier and only occasionally in later years. Second, it doesn't always, or even often, include tendencies toward violence. Schizophrenia is one of society's most misunderstood conditions, one that people tend to fear in others, and one that retains stigma even as we make progress destigmatizing other conditions such as anxiety and bipolar depression. I mention this here because we have already seen that Richard Dadd's form of schizophrenia was violent, and we're about to see that this is true of Louis Wain as well. The stories of their lives should not be misinterpreted to indicate that schizophrenia causes people to commit violent acts. In fact, due to the vulnerability of their condition, **people with schizophrenia are far more likely to be a victim of a crime than they are to perpetrate one.**[2] Some modern psychologists even argue that we need a new category of mental health classification specifically for schizophrenic symptoms with aggressive, hostile, and violent tendencies.[3] Unfortunately, rare though it is, Louis Wain is another example of an artist with a violent manifestation of schizophrenia.

Louis Wain acts almost as a "poster child" for this disorder as it relates to creativity; he is frequently cited as someone whose artwork shows a clear progression of the condition. If you want to learn about an artist whose perception was affected by schizophrenia, your preliminary research will almost always turn up Wain as a source.[4]

Schizophrenia, like any mental health condition, manifests and progresses differently in individual people, so to say one person's journey is the quintessential example of a condition is a falsehood in any case. Furthermore, Wain wouldn't really be the ideal example of the "normal" presentation of the illness.

Before falling ill, Wain was already a successful artist, making his living as an illustrator.[5] He is said to have illustrated more than two hundred books that sold prolifically.[6] He created thousands of cartoons and illustrations, which were published in children's magazines as well as in his own annual publication.[7]

But in 1924, Wain was checked into a psychiatric asylum after exhibiting symptoms of violence, particularly aggression toward at least one of his sisters.[8] He was already sixty-four years old, very unusually late in life for schizophrenia to develop, but this is the best diagnosis we have today to fit the available information. Louis Wain was very physically ill at a young age and didn't start attending school until he was ten, which stunted him socially.[9] Later, he would struggle financially and lose the love of his life to illness, all traumas that may have helped trigger his symptoms.

Wain is most famous for his images of cats, specifically cats that are performing human tasks, such as golfing or sitting at a table drinking tea. As mentioned in the chapter on Richard Dadd, some asylums in the nineteenth century attempted to provide a range of therapeutic services to the patients. In addition to art, keeping animals as pets was a form of therapy being explored during this time. When Louis Wain was at Napsbury Hospital, it had a garden with cats, which proved to be a blessing.[10] Napsbury was a big improvement for Wain, who had first been imprisoned at Springfield Mental Hospital, where even when he was lucid he did not have access to paper and pencil to sketch.[11] Luckily, several people intervened on his behalf to get him transferred to better facilities where he was allowed to make his art, and where some say he produced his best work, though it differed greatly from his previous style.[12] A doctor at Bedlam noted of this change: "His executive technique has largely disintegrated. He is at present . . . a man of fantastic delusions."[13]

Wain was obviously a cat lover. He adored them, and cats were the subject he most often illustrated. As one author describes, while his wife, Emily, "was gradually succumbing to illness over a period of several years, Wain often used the household cat, Peter, to amuse her, dressing him up in glasses and making it seem as if he were reading the paper, just for chuckles."[14] Wain and Emily were married in 1884, but she passed away only three years later and he never remarried. Wain grew close with the cat that he had used to cheer his wife during her illness, and in an 1886 piece of writing, he extolled the therapeutic benefits of keeping cats as pets.[15] It seemed that having the cat assisted him through the deep sadness of losing his wife. Peter was his companion for another decade, but Wain was devastated when he eventually passed away. Wain's grief manifested in depression and anxiety, and he struggled to make a living as an artist.[16] Things got worse during World War I, when there was a paper shortage, making it hard for him to find buyers for his illustrations. He needed to support his mother and five sisters, but by the 1920s he was impoverished, the stress of which may have exacerbated his symptoms.[17]

As Wain began to lost touch with reality, affinity for cats became more complex and obsessive. He said that cats "accursed him" and "robbed him of his wealth, his health and his reason."[18] In the early 1900s he began to write about the idea that cats, too, can have mental illness, saying, "Cats are often driven mad or imbecile by excessive punishment or fright."[19] In 1914 Wain fell off an omnibus and hit his head, becoming concussed. (Ironically, the omnibus swerved to avoid hitting a cat—though this is alleged and may be posthumous mythologizing of the role that cats played in Wain's mental deterioration.[20]) In any case, his sisters believed this head injury to be the source of or trigger for their brother's madness, and from this point on he became increasingly violent, especially acting out against his sister Claire. This violence was what ultimately led to his institutionalization when his sisters had him committed.[21]

Thankfully, Wain's violence never rose to the homicidal degree of Richard Dadd, but it was certainly enough of a problem to be of concern. Author Paul Moody shares the following:

> The prospect of having to produce yet more pictures took a heavy toll on a psyche already damaged by the death of his sister Marie in an asylum two years previously. The final straw came with the death of another sister, Caroline, in 1917. Wain became neurotic and obsessed with order, rearranging the furniture in the family's house in Kilburn, sometimes on an hourly basis. Prone to paranoid delusions, and believing that his remaining sisters were plotting to kill him, he tried to throw one of them down the stairs before the family reluctantly had him certified insane in June 1924.[22]

Discussing his violent actions with doctors, Wain said irrational things, such as "the electricity of the cinema has taken the electricity out of his sisters' brains."[23] He became increasingly suspicious, thinking that people were robbing him, and that there was ether in his food.[24] Modern psychiatrist Dr. David O'Flynn points out that the artist was exhibiting signs of thought disorder as early as 1910, as evidenced by his own writings, which exhibited a broken-down language structure, a symptom primarily associated with schizophrenia.[25] So, the condition may have manifested much earlier than originally thought.

Many have theorized that you can look at the progression of Wain's art, from the earliest cat paintings to the last, and see a clear and steady disintegration of style as he further fell into the depths of schizophrenia. Writer Silvia Helena Cardosa describes:

> Quite revealing of his psychotic condition were the cat's eyes. See how they become fixed with hostility, even in the earliest paintings, because the psychotic probably tends to think that the world is looking upon him in a menacing way. Another sign is the fragmentation of the cat's body.[26]

Joseph Milton notes of Wain's cats that they "became more abstract until, towards the end of his life, they were barely recognisable as cats at all, instead becoming intricately detailed, fractal shapes full of unnaturally (at least for a cat) bright colours."[27] However, this "timeline" of his creations has more recently been contested. Author Paul Gallagher tells us that "though it is believed that Louis Wain's paintings followed a direct line towards schizophrenia, it is unknown in which order Wain made his pictures. Like his finances, Wain's mental state was erratic throughout his life, which may explain the changes back and forth between the cute and cuddly and the abstract and psychedelic."[28] We might be able to attribute the idea that his work was created in a certain order, showing a linear progression of the disease, to psychiatrist Dr. Walter Maclay, who "discovered" Wain's work in 1939 and held an exhibition of it at Bethlem Museum of the Mind, located at the Bethlem Royal Hospital, where Wain was a patient for several years. He made the decision to order the works in a format that showed mental deterioration, but he may have taken too much creative license with the linear timeline.[29] Here we see the problematic side of "outsider art" appreciation, in which interpretations of the art are skewed to fit a predetermined narrative.

In truth, Wain's mental health fluctuated and did not simply diminish in an ever-disintegrating line.

In 1928, Louis Wain created a powerful sketch of a happy-looking cat with text underneath that reads "I am happy because everyone loves me," which seems to indicate a positive mental state. Then again, at Bedlam he reportedly at times refused to bathe and would drink paraffin whenever he could sneak it.[30] By the following year, a note in the same chart says that he had gotten calmer, suggesting a nonlinear progression of his disease rather than a clear descension from "healthy" to "crazy." Mental illness is rarely neat or predictable. Although his work is not likely an exact representation of his illness, it does in some way provide insight into his psychological state. One critic posits that "images are fingerprints of the mind; the architecture of the mind encodes itself in representational form, whether we're trying to render that or not."[31]

Cats make up a huge part of the artist's subject matter throughout his lifetime. This was initially because they became known as his signature, and it was profitable to stick with the theme. But recall from the chapter on Richard Dadd that repetition of themes is common in art produced by people with schizophrenia. The repetition compulsion is strong across many artists but is particularly common in those with a schizophrenic spectrum diagnosis. Some argue that **artwork can even be used as a diagnostic tool** to determine whether or not a patient has schizophrenia.[32] It's not necessarily the technique that differs between so-called "normal" art and the art of schizophrenia, but rather the content. Other than repetition, some of the commonalities include "desexualized figures, strong border lines, symmetry, and especially misidentification and fusion of objects or figures."[33] Recognizing these patterns allows therapists to better understand what's going on in the patient's mind. The patient uses the art to attempt to express their experience of reality, a process that can actually help build self-esteem for the artist with schizophrenia.[34]

Wain produced art both before and after his time in the asylum, and his style changed drastically during his mental health journey. He had an almost single minded interest in cats, which became an important and repetitive theme in his art, as well as a tool for therapy in his treatment at the asylum. He shows us how something that can be good for the mind—whether that's a fixation with animals or life as an artist—can also become a source of angst or trouble. When Wain's cats devolve into abstraction, becoming just lines and colors, mere suggestions of cats, was it due to the symptoms of his mental health challenges? Or is it simply a creative evolution? The two cannot really be separated.

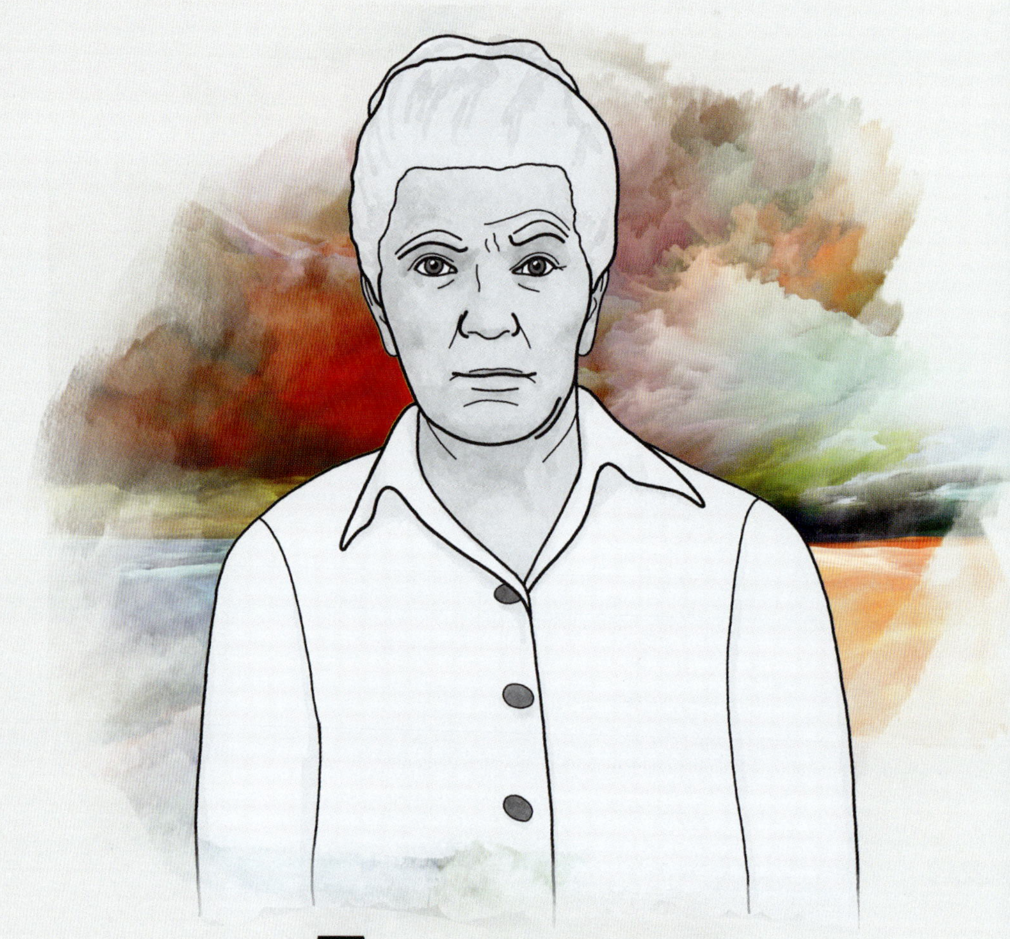

Aloïse Corbaz

(June 28, 1886–April 5, 1964)

O sorrow! O despair! I never managed to seize the delicate flowers and their penetrating perfumes that you were involuntarily depositing in each corner of my heart immured by misery. That [I can] not requench my blazing soul.

–ALOÏSE CORBAZ, LETTER TO GUILLAUME II[1]

Aloïse Corbaz worked as a teacher and governess at the court of German kaiser Wilhelm II, during which time she developed what's been called an "obsessive romantic passion" for him.[2] There are no indications, however, that they ever had any actual romantic connection other than in her mind.[3] Although Corbaz left the court and returned to her home in Switzerland at the start of World War II, she apparently remained fixated on the emperor and believed that she and Kaiser Wilhelm II were continuing their passionate love affair. Ultimately, this delusion led to the diagnosis of schizophrenia, for which she was institutionalized at La Rosière asylum in Gimel.[4]

Corbaz became a prolific artist and writer during her time in the institution, although it took time for her doctors to understand the importance of her creativity to her mental health. She was institutionalized in 1918, and for years her sketches and writings on various scraps of paper were dismissed as the products of a "mad woman." For this reason, many of her early works were destroyed. Finally, though, in 1936, Dr. Jaqueline Porret-Forel began to interpret the writings as poetry, instead of as delusional ramblings.[5] After convincing asylum manager Hans Steck of this idea, they began to offer Aloïse access to large sheets of paper on which to write and draw.[6] She still sometimes used discarded sheets of paper, gift wrap, and cardboard stitched together to create even-larger works.[7] Corbaz worked with whatever medium she could get her hands on, including chalk, gouache, and even toothpaste and crushed flower petals.[8]

Initially, she did a lot of romantic writing expressing her continuing delusions of nonexistent relationships, illustrating them with colored pencils. That theme would be continued over the course of her life, but Corbaz's work progressed with time, and she began to use bolder, less "romantic" colors, along with striking compositional choices.[9] In later pieces, although a couple was often the centerpiece of an image, she would also add other figures (women, children, and even symbolic figures such as popes), nature, animals, and vehicles.[10] Even these other details, though, were typically meant to be autobiographical. Dr. Porret-Forel says, "She was never happier than when the flower or animal that she had just drawn represented her."[11] Using animals and other figures as stand-ins for the self brings to mind the work of Leonora Carrington, another artist who experienced delusions, and begs the question if these metaphorical connections are made in part because of the disordered ways in which these artists' minds were working.

In addition to her drawings, Corbaz's writings can also be considered as visual art. Author Jina Valentine argues that reading transcribed versions of her textual work misses the point because it's in the visual depiction that the meaning emerges. Examples she gives of artistic decisions that Corbaz makes in these works are single words taking up entire lines, words darkened or retraced for emphasis, serifs of letters used to underline words, capitalization, writing in all directions, and adding images to text.[12] She adds, "The revisions, effacings, and creases are signs that writing took place over the course of multiple sessions, and that the papers were carried around in between," which implies that these works held the same importance for Corbaz as any of her pictorial pieces.[13] She also points out that some of the decisions about the way text was placed on the page could have been due, at least in part, to limitations in her access to material. Her work would have been entirely different if she'd "recorded her sentiments on a typewriter, or written on pristine, lined paper."[14] Society tends to think of text works as being a form of communication to the reader, but perhaps in Corbaz's case it was not. Valentine posits that she did her writing and her art for herself, not for anyone else, which is one of the most widely admired defining aspects of so-called outsider art.

About ten years after the asylum began to encourage Corbaz's creativity, her artwork was "discovered" by artist Jean Dubuffet, who included her in his initial research into "art brut" or outsider art.[15]

Despite the fact that her romantic delusions continued, Dubuffet expressed the belief that the artist had actually cured herself of madness by choosing not to fight it but instead to give into it completely, allowing her delusions (and the art she created as a result) to become her reason to live.[16] Dr. Porret-Forel presents a slightly different but not altogether dissenting idea: that Corbaz, unable to live within the chaos of the "real" world, created her own reality, a "cosmogonic theater," or "a supernatural world, theater of the Universe" in which she was able to thrive.[17] Aloïse Corbaz herself stated that art was her "only source of perpetual ecstasy." This sentiment could be applied to any of the artists in this book and may be at the crux of why art is often so important to those with mental illness.

In recent years, with growing research into the neurochemistry of schizophrenia, many have wondered whether or not Corbaz would have been able to create the art she did if she existed in a modern-day society, where people are often medicated for the condition. Research indicates that people with schizophrenia may have low levels of dopamine receptors, which allows for unusual creative connections; they see and experience things that people with higher dopamine levels do not, and this can come through in artistic expression.[18] If that's the case, then the medication that helps treat schizophrenia may also remove some of these connections. Some argue that were Aloïse alive today and medicated, she would be able to live freely outside an institution—but perhaps at a cost to her art.[19]

If art was a retreat or balm for Corbaz, would she be satisfied having medication as an alternative treatment? Or would she have missed out on the "ecstasy of life" that she experienced as a direct result of her creative process? As one author living with schizophrenia notes, "She would not have had the protective and safe environment in which her art would thrive and flourish. She was allowed a total of 46 years['] work with her illness in safety through the creative arts."[20] The situation calls to mind Yayoi Kusama, who also experienced hallucinations and has had a thriving art career while choosing to live for decades in the insular and structured setting of a psychiatric institution.

Once admitted to the asylum, Corbaz remained there for more than forty years, dying while still institutionalized at close to eighty years old. She has more than two thousand works of art that have been collected into an online catalogue raisonne by Porret-Forel, the doctor who worked with her artistically in the asylum and who has been a lifelong champion of her work.[21] For what it's worth, the doctor has said that although she believes in the value of medication to relieve people from their mental suffering, she also agrees that Corbaz would have been an entirely different type of artist, perhaps not becoming one at all, had antipsychotic medication been available to her during her lifetime.[22] Again we see art making itself as a medicine of sorts, allowing Corbaz a joyful and productive life within the confines of her mental illness.

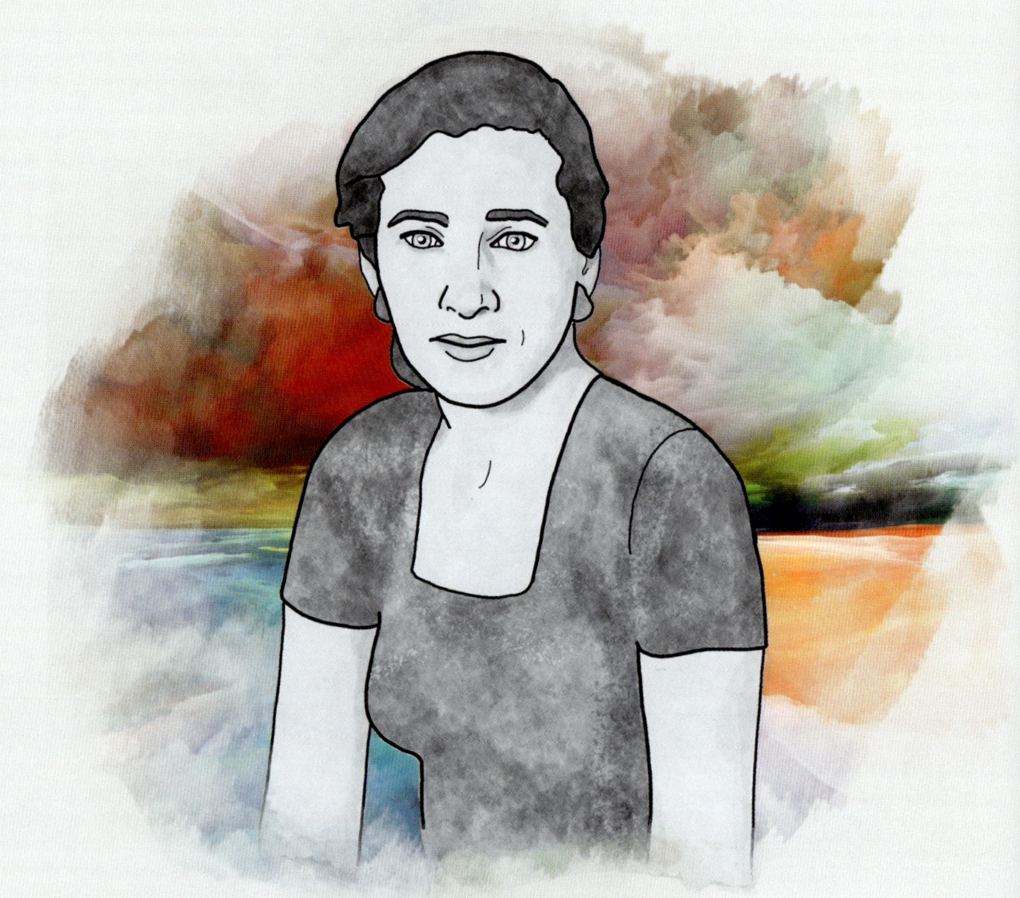

Agnes Martin

(March 22, 1912–December 16, 2004)

The silence on the floor of my house
Is all the questions and all the answers that have been known in the world
The sentimental furniture threatens the peace
The reflection of a sunset speaks loudly of days

—AGNES MARTIN[1]

Agnes Martin is an important figure in art history and is still sometimes included in lists of "outsider artists." We include her here to further emphasize the arbitrary nature of the term. Martin had a diagnosis of schizophrenia and spent time in institutions but managed to conceal her diagnosis from the public for ninety-plus years. She was arguably "outside" mainstream culture in other ways, as a Canadian-born lesbian who left New York City, the center of the art world universe, to instead live in solitude in New Mexico. However, she was also represented by the Betty Parsons Gallery and by Pace Gallery's Arne Glimcher. She was employed as an art teacher and was friends and acquaintances with countless other artists and art professionals. It was not as if she was unaware of or separate from the important goings-on of the mainstream art world. In fact, she played a critical role in the stylistic progression from abstract expressionism to minimalism, which can't be understated in the history of art. As her biographer Nancy Princenthal puts it: "I'm leery of sweeping her up in this celebration of artists, these artists who are self-trained or outsider, or beyond the pale of cosmopolitan art and life, and that's their merit. I think her mental illness is liable to enforce that impulse and I think that would be a mistake."[2] This is not to say we should ignore Martin's mental health. Like Yayoi Kusama, her struggles are integral to the body of work she created. **Perhaps what we can learn best from Martin is how one can find a path forward when facing mental health issues.**

People have frequently emphasized Agnes Martin's preference for solitude and her tendency to emotionally distance herself from others. We can perhaps look to her early childhood to understand why this might be. Agnes Martin's father died when she was just two years old, so she was raised primarily by a single mother, Margaret, with help from Agnes's maternal grandfather.[3] Martin's mother has been called a "hard" woman. There's a story that when Agnes was only six years old, she reportedly had tonsillitis, so her mother gave her some money to take the streetcar to the hospital. The young Martin went by herself to have the operation and returned home the same way.[4] Martin was close with her maternal grandfather, but that relationship was also described as distanced—more intellectual than warm and loving.[5]

Martin took a series of odd jobs in her teens and twenties, ranging from ice cream packer to juvenile warden, and ultimately landed in a position in New York teaching art. Martin quickly decided, around the age of thirty, that she wanted a career as an artist herself.[6] After spending some time working in New York, she—like Georgia O'Keeffe—escaped to the quiet deserts of New Mexico. In 1955, with a grant from the Helene Wurlitzer Foundation, she created over a hundred paintings in a single year.[7] In the late 1950s she met art dealer Betty Parsons, who agreed to represent her, but only if she would move back to New York City, and so she did.[8]

Although Martin was able to keep her diagnosis of schizophrenia secret from the world until after her death at the age of ninety-two, she struggled with the symptoms, particularly extensive confusion and emotional dysregulation, and required hospitalization.[9] She had auditory hallucinations throughout her life, was in and out of hospitals for treatment, and tried both medication and talk therapy for healing.[10] During one spell when she didn't know who she was and was found wandering around New York, Martin was sent to Bellevue (the same psychiatric hospital Yayoi Kusama spent time in when she lived in New York). While there, Martin was treated with electroshock therapy, which may have affected her memory for the rest of her life.[11] In addition to her hallucinations, Martin experienced periods of depression, sometimes to the point of catatonia, which includes symptoms of not speaking and of staying still for long periods of time. Moreover, she was intensely sensitive to music, citing one time that three notes into a Bach song at a church she fell into a catatonic state.[12] People with catatonic depression often appear as if they are dazed or unresponsive.

After about ten years in New York City, Martin experienced a series of difficulties that put a pause to her art making: she and her girlfriend broke up, the building she lived in was torn down, and her close friend and fellow artist Ad Reinhardt passed away.[13] Martin's mental health was suffering. She needed a change, so she gave away her art supplies, loaded herself into a truck, and spent two years traveling, living mostly in trailer parks, until finally landing back in New Mexico and making it her permanent home.[14] Reportedly, she experienced a vision that told her to go back to the southwestern state.[15] She didn't paint at all during those two years, and it took another five before she began making art again.[16] Although this was the longest break Martin took from painting, there was an ebb and flow to her work that included times of not producing much at all, a pattern that perhaps coincided with her mental health. After months with no inspiration to paint, Martin would begin again and, very slowly and gradually, gain creative steam again.[17]

To validate her own experience, Agnes Martin was very clear that she did not see her art as having anything at all to do with her mental illness.[18] Yet, her biographer notes that the way in which Martin spoke of her paintings coming to her as fully formed visions hints at symptoms of her mental health issues.[19] Princenthal ultimately concludes that Martin's work was meant to represent the universal, not the personal, and should not be viewed as catharsis or some form of art therapy for her schizophrenia.[20]

Still, others have suggested that the minimalist nature of Martin's work, the straight lines and grids, is a reflection of **an attempt to give order to her own mental chaos**. Martin was once quoted as saying, "Into my mind there came a grid, and it looked like innocence."[21] She also once wrote, "My formats are square but the grids never are absolutely square; they are rectangles, a little bit off the square, making a sort of contradiction, a dissonance. . . . When I cover the square surface with rectangles, it lightens the weight of the square, destroys its power."[22] Though we agree with Princenthal that Martin's work should not be solely read as some kind art therapy, it does seem as though **painting served a therapeutic**

purpose for her, helping her make sense of the world and to work through her issues. We know that Martin was quite spiritual, with a specific interest in the philosophy of Zen Buddhism, and she did regard her creative practice as a form of meditation, a way to let go of the ego and tap into the sublime.[23] Journalist Olivia Laing writes of Martin's work that "these images of absolute calm did not arise from a life replete with love or ease, but rather out of turbulence, solitude and hardship. Though inspired, they represent an act of dogged will and extreme effort, and their perfection is hard-won."[24]

The land of New Mexico was a home she chose for its quietude, and so one has to ask if her choices to live an often-isolated life had anything to do with her schizophrenia. Biographer Nancy Princenthal shares that there are different clusters of symptoms within schizophrenia, one of which includes social withdrawal, along with apathy and other "negative" symptoms. She goes on to argue that Martin's withdrawal, combined with the almost ascetic way of life she imposed upon herself, and the "formalized nature of her conversations" are all indicative of this cluster of symptoms, an argument supported by psychiatrist Mark Epstein.[25] Although Epstein agrees with the likelihood of her diagnosis of schizophrenia, he also notes that her high levels of productivity between episodes suggest that it's possible she had schizoaffective disorder, or perhaps even bipolar disorder.[26] As we saw in the chapter on Edvard Munch, there's much overlap among these symptoms, making it hard to fully distinguish one from the other.

Martin, who continued working up until the time that she passed away—approximately sixty years after starting her art career—notoriously valued her privacy, even to the detriment of her own legacy. As journalist Carolina A. Miranda describes: "She destroyed early works, actively discouraged the publication of monographs about her art[,] and made friends swear that they wouldn't talk about her after her death."[27] Although she would later give many talks, and she would share her thoughts through prolific writing, she didn't particularly like to be interviewed, once telling an interviewer that being on his tape recorder would give him too much power.[28] Maybe her tendency toward privacy was because of the stigma associated with schizophrenia; she didn't want others to know that she struggled with this condition. Perhaps it was because of the stigma of being a member of the LGBTQIA+ community. Or perhaps it was just the nature of her own personality. But her fierce privacy forces us to ask what right or role *we* as outsiders have bringing our own interpretations to her work. And it's an important reminder that while there might be value for both art and psychology to explore an artist's work through the lens of mental health, we also always do so through the lenses of our own biases.

NOTES

INTRODUCTION

1. Jane Kromm, "Psychological States and the Artist: The Problem of Michelangelo," *Studies in Visual Communication* 6, no. 1 (1980): 72.
2. Katherine Williams, *Women on the Verge: The Culture of Neurasthenia in Nineteenth-Century America* (Stanford, CA: Iris & B. Gerald Cantor Center for Visual Arts at Stanford University, 2004), 1.
3. Ibid.
4. Ibid., 7.
5. Ibid.

I. ART'S "MAD GENIUS": VINCENT VAN GOGH

1. Vincent van Gogh, *Ever Yours: The Essential Letters*, ed. Leo Jansen, Hans Luijten, and Nienke Bakker (New Haven, CT: Yale University Press, 2014), 73.
2. Dietrich Blumer, "The Illness of Vincent Van Gogh," *American Journal of Psychiatry* 159, no. 4 (April 2002): 519.
3. Dean Keith Simonton, "Are Genius and Madness Related? Contemporary Answers to an Ancient Question," *Psychiatric Times* 22, no. 7 (May 2005).
4. Arne Dietrich, "The Mythconception of the Mad Genius," *Frontiers in Psychology*, February 2014.
5. Simonton, "Are Genius and Madness Related?"
6. Ibid.
7. Ibid.
8. Dietrich, "The Mythconception of the Mad Genius."
9. Kalyan B. Bhattacharyya and Saurabh Rai, "The Neuropsychiatric Ailment of Vincent Van Gogh," *Annals of Indian Academy of Neurology* 18, no. 1 (2015): 6-9.
10. Martin Bailey, *Starry Night: Van Gogh at the Asylum* (London: White Lion, 2018).
11. Craig Wright, "Is There a Thin Line between Genius and Insanity?," *Psychology Today*, 2020.
12. Ibid.
13. Jonathan Jones, "Vincent Van Gogh: Myths, Madness and a New Way of Painting," *Guardian*, August 5, 2016.
14. Ibid.
15. Ibid.
16. Wright, "Is There a Thin Line between Genius and Insanity?"
17. Ibid.

18. Maria Popova, "Van Gogh and Mental Illness," Brain Pickings, March 30, 2017.
19. Jones, "Vincent Van Gogh: Myths, Madness and a New Way of Painting."
20. Ibid.
21. Sarah Cascone, "Doctors Cannot Figure Out Vincent Van Gogh's Illness," Artnet News, September 17, 2016.
22. Blumer, "The Illness of Vincent Van Gogh," 519.

II. CREATING IN DARKNESS: ARTISTS WITH DEPRESSION SPECTRUM DISORDERS

1. "Any Mood Disorder," 2017, National Institute of Mental Health, US Department of Health and Human Services, nimh.nih.gov.

MICHELANGELO BUONARROTI

1. Lewis, J. Patrick, and Michelangelo Buonarroti, *Michelangelo's World* (Mankato, MN: Creative Editions, 2007), 6.
2. Ibid., 70.
3. Barbara A. Somervill, *Michelangelo: Sculptor and Painter* (Minneapolis, MN: Capstone, 2008), 15.
4. Ibid.
5. Anthony Storr, *Solitude: A Return to the Self* (New York: Simon and Schuster, 2005), 138.
6. Ross King, *Michelangelo & the Pope's Ceiling* (London: Penguin Books, 2003), 195-196.
7. Crompton, 272.
8. James M. Saslow, "James M. Saslow on Sensuality and Spirituality in Michelangelo's Poetry," metmuseum.org, 2018.
9. Ibid., 269.
10. Ibid., 270.
11. Somervill, 85.
12. Jane Kristof, "Michelangelo as Nicodemus: The Florence Pieta," *The Sixteenth Century Journal* 20, no. 2 (1989): pp. 163-182, 169.
13. Martin Gayford, *Michelangelo: His Epic Life* (London: Penguin UK, 2013).
14. Somervill, 10.
15. Gayford.
16. Somervill, 10.
17. Ibid., 9.
18. Kromm, 71.
19. Somervill, 10.
20. Michelangelo, *Complete Poems of Michelangelo*, trans. John Frederick Nims (Chicago, IL: University of Chicago Press, 2000), 169.

21. Ibid., 17.
22. Gayford.
23. Kromm, 71.

FRANCISCO GOYA

1. Larry Chang, *Wisdom for the Soul: Five Millennia of Prescriptions for Spiritual Healing* (Washington, DC: Gnosophia Publishers, 2006), 384.
2. D. Felisati and G. Sperati, "Francisco Goya and His Illness," *Acta Otorhinolaryngologica Italica: Organo Ufficiale Della Società Italiana Di Otorinolaringologia e Chirurgia Cervico-Facciale* 30 (October 5, 2010): pp. 264-270.
3. Tugce Toptan, et al. "Neurosyphilis: a Case Report," *Northern Clinics of Istanbul* 2, no. 1 (2015): pp. 66-68.
4. Felisati.
5. Ibid.
6. Alan E.H. Henry, "The Madhouse by Francisco Goya," *Practical Neurology* 3 (2003): pp. 178-183.
7. Laura L. Casey, "Goya: 'In Sickness and in Health'," *International Journal of Surgery* 4, no. 1 (2006): pp. 66-72. https://doi.org/10.1016/j.ijsu.2005.08.001.
8. Robert Hughes, *Goya* (New York: Knopf Doubleday Publishing Group, 2012).
9. Ibid.
10. Ibid.
11. Amy Novotney, "The Risks of Social Isolation," *Monitor on Psychology* 50, no. 5 (2019): p. 32.
12. Casey.
13. Klein, 198.
14. Ibid.

DISABILITY & ILLNESS

1. R. Jay Turner and Samuel Noh, "Physical Disability and Depression: A Longitudinal Analysis," *Journal of Health and Social Behavior* 29, no. 1 (1988): p. 23, https://doi.org/10.2307/2137178.
2. Jennifer Sullivan Sulewski, Heike Boeltzig, and Rooshey Hasnain, "Art and Disability: Intersecting Identities among Young Artists with Disabilities," *Disability Studies Quarterly* 32, no. 1 (2012), https://doi.org/10.18061/dsq.v32i1.3034.

EDVARD MUNCH

1. Sue Prideaux, *Edvard Munch: Behind The Scream* (New Haven, CT: Yale University Press, 2019), 251.
2. Ibid., 210.

3. Demitri F. Papolos and Janice Papolos, *The Bipolar Child (Third Edition): The Definitive and Reassuring Guide to Childhood's Most Misunderstood Disorder* (New York: Broadway Books, 2006), 216.
4. Albert Rothenberg, "Bipolar Illness, Creativity, and Treatment," *Psychiatric Quarterly* 72, no. 2 (2001): pp. 131-147, 137.
5. Hina Azeem, "The Art of Edvard Munch: A Window Onto a Mind," *BJPsych Advances* 21, no. 1 (2015): pp. 51-53, 51.
6. Sophia Beams, "The Scream: A Deeper Analysis of Edvard Munch's Anxiety-Wrought Piece," Medium.com (Everything Art, August 2, 2019).
7. Jon Mann, "How Edvard Munch Expressed the Anxiety of the Modern World," Artsy.net, July 10, 2017.
8. Ibid.
9. Andreas Ebert and Karl-Jürgen Bär, "Emil Kraepelin: A Pioneer of Scientific Understanding of Psychiatry and Psychopharmacology," *Indian Journal of Psychiatry* 52, no. 2 (April 2010): pp. 191-192, 191.
10. Ibid., 192.
11. Adrian Preda, MD. "The Difference Between Schizophrenia and Schizoaffective Disorder." Verywell Mind, January 31, 2020.
12. Prideaux, 228.
13. Ibid.
14. Ibid.
15. Ibid.
16. Azeem, 51.
17. Ibid.
18. Knausgård.
19. Azeem, 52.
20. James C. Harris, "Art and Images in Psychiatry," *Archives of General Psychiatry* 64, no. 9 (2007): pp. 996-997.
21. Ibid.
22. Harris, 997.
23. Lubow.
24. Ibid.
25. Ibid.
26. Ibid.
27. Ibid.
28. Ibid.
29. Prideaux, 241.
30. Azeem, 53.
31. Prideaux, 246-250.
32. Rothenberg, 145.
33. Vladimir Maletic, "Differentiating Between Bipolar and Schizoaffective Diagnoses," Psychiatry & Behavioral Health Learning Network, March 6, 2020, psychcongress.com
34. Rothenberg, 137.
35. Prideaux, 246-250.
36. Ibid., 251.
37. Azeem, 53.
38. Ibid., 53.
39. Ibid.
40. Knausgaard.

41. Beams.
42. Ibid.
43. Rothenberg
44. Mann.

INFLUENCE ON CONTEMPORARY ARTISTS: TRACEY EMIN

1. Jennifer Higgie, "Tracey Emin's Lifelong Affinity with Edvard Munch" (Royal Academy of Arts, November 30, 2020), https://www.royalacademy.org.uk/article/tracey-emin-jennifer-higgie-interview.
2. Rosemary Waugh, "The Enduring Connection between Art and Mental Health" (Art UK, November 4, 2020), https://artuk.org/discover/stories/e-enduring-connection-between-art-and-mental-health.

GEORGIA O'KEEFFE

1. Olivia Laing, "The Wild Beauty of Georgia O'Keeffe," *Guardian* (Guardian News and Media, July 1, 2016).
2. "Facts & Statistics," Anxiety and Depression Association of America, ADAA.org.
3. Udall, 17
4. Laing.
5. Ibid.
6. Ibid.
7. Ibid.
8. Arlin Cuncic, "What High Functioning Anxiety Feels Like," Verywell Mind, May 11, 2020, https://www.verywellmind.com/what-is-high-functioning-anxiety-4140198.
9. Udall,18
10. Laing.
11. Ibid,18.
12. Ibid,19.
13. Ibid.
14. Ibid., 20.
15. Ibid.
16. Laing.
17. Udall, 21.
18. Popova.
19. Lisa Messinger, "Georgia O'Keeffe (1887-1986)," metmuseum.org, 2004, https://www.metmuseum.org/toah/hd/geok/hd_geok.htm.

JOAN MIRÓ

1. Joseph J. Schildkraut, "Opinion: Miró Offers Case in Point of

Creativity's Link to Depression," *New York Times*, 1993, sec. 4, p. 14.
2. Ibid.
3. Schildkraut.
4. Montserrat G. Delgado and Julien Bogousslavsky, "Joan Miró and Cyclic Depression," *Frontiers of Neurology and Neuroscience* 43 (2018): pp. 1-7, https://doi.org/10.1159/000490400.
5. Bogousslavsky and Tatu.
6. Michael Kimmelman, "The Creative Mind Reader," *New York Times*, December 31, 2006, National edition, sec. 6, p. 12, https://www.nytimes.com/2006/12/31/magazine/the-creative-mind-reader.html.
7. Stanley Meisler, "For Joan Miró, Poetry and Painting Were the Same," *Smithsonian Magazine*, November 1993, http://www.stanleymeisler.com/smithsonian/smithsonian-1993-11-Miro.html.
8. John Canaday, "Calder and Miró; One's Mobiles, the Other's Paintings, In a Just About Perfect Show," *New York Times*, February 26, 1961, sec. X, p. 19, https://www. nytimes.com/1961/02/26/archives/calder-and-Miró-onesmobiles-the-others-paintings-in-a-just-about.html.
9. Miró, Lubar, and Tailandier.
10. Meisler.
11. Ibid.
12. Meisler.
13. Michael Gibson, "An Uneasy Stroll through Early Miró," *International Herald Tribune*, March 6, 2004, https://www.nytimes.com/2004/03/06/style/an-uneasy-stroll-throughearly-mir.html.
14. Richardson.
15. Meisler.
16. Delgado and Bogousslavsky.
17. Kimmelman.
18. Ibid.
19. Miró, Lubar, and Tailandier, 11.
20. Ibid.
21. Delgado and Bogousslavsky.
22. Ibid.
23. Maria Popova, "I Work Like a Gardener: Joan Miró on Art, Motionless Movement, and the Proper Pace of Creative Labor," Brain Pickings, September 18, 2018, https://www. brainpickings.org/2015/09/17/i-work-like-a-gardener-joan-miro/.

ALICE NEEL

1. Phoebe Hoban, *Alice Neel: The Art of Not Sitting Pretty* (New York: St. Martin's, 2010), 79.
2. Kennaugh, Stuart. "Biography." Alice Neel. Accessed July 30, 2020. http://www.aliceneel.com/biography/.
3. Kennaugh.
4. Maine, Stephen. "Thriving on Drama and Discordance: The Life of Alice Neel." artcritical, August 3, 2011. https://artcritical.com/2011

/08/02/alice-neel/.
5. Kennaugh.
6. Bridget Quinn and Lisa Congdon, *Broad Strokes: 15 Women Who Made Art and Made History (in That Order)* (San Francisco, CA: Chronicle Books, 2017), 105.
7. Grace Glueck, "Alice Neel, Self-Styled 'Collector of Souls,' Unfurls Her Own, in Glee and Heartbreak," *New York Times*, March 21, 1997, National edition, sec. C, p. 25
8. Denise Bauer, "Alice Neel's Portraits of Mother Work," *NWSA Journal* 14, no. 2 (2002): 108
9. Ibid., 77.
10. Kennaugh.
11. Hoban, 79.
12. Helen Harrison, "Art; Catching Corners of the Human Spirit," *New York Times*, May 4, 1986, National edition, sec. 11LI, p. 32.
13. Ibid.
14. Kennaugh.
15. Ibid. (Millet refused, as she believed not one person could or should represent the cause, and Neel had to work from photographs.)
16. Glueck.
17. Ibid.
18. Anthony John Febles, "Rosenbergs Remembered in Sympathetic Exhibit," Daily Collegian, March 24, 1989, www.collegian.psu.edu.

ARTISTS AND SUICIDE

1. Nancy C. Andreasen, "The Relationship Between Creativity and Mood Disorders," *Dialogues in Clinical Neuroscience* 10, no. 2 (2008): pp. 251-255, https://doi.org/10.31887/dcns.2008.10.2/ncandreasen.
2. Ewan Morrison, "The Suicidal Artist," *Psychology Today* (Sussex Publishers, April 2, 2019), https://www.psychologytoday.com/us/blog/word-less/201904/the-suicidal-artist.
3. Jill Sonke et al., "Systematic Review of Arts-Based Interventions to Address Suicide Prevention and Survivorship in Australia, Canada, the United Kingdom, and the United States of America," *Health Promotion Practice* 22, no. 1_suppl (2021), https://doi.org/10.1177/1524839921996350.

MARK ROTHKO

1. Edward Alden Jewell, "'Globalism' Pops Into View," *New York Times*, June 13, 1943, p. 219.
2. Lee Seldes, *The Legacy of Mark Rothko* (New York: Da Capo Press, 1996), 10-11.
3. Seldes, 11.
4. Hartman JJ, "Risk Factors in Suicide: Mark Rothko and His Art," *Journal of Psychiatry and Mental Health* 3, no. 2 (2018), https://doi.org/10.16966/2474-7769.127, 2.

5. Cohen-Solal.
6. Seldes, 13.
7. "Artist Mark Rothko," American Masters Podcast (PBS, October 29, 2019).
8. Grace Glueck, "Mark Rothko, Artist, A Suicide Here at 66," *New York Times*, February 26, 1970, p. 1, https://www. nytimes.com/1970/02/26/archives/mark-rothko-artist-a-suicide-here-at-66-mark-rothko-abstract.html.
9. Ibid., 16.
10. Ibid.
11. Seldes, 13.
12. James E. B. Breslin, *Mark Rothko: a Biography* (Chicago, IL: University of Chicago Press, 1998), 169-170.
13. Breslin, 240.
14. Glueck.
15. Ibid.
16. Breslin, 265.
17. Breslin, 286.
18. JJ, 3.
19. Hilarie M. Sheets, "Mark Rothko's Dark Palette Illuminated," *New York Times*, November 3, 2016, sec. C, p. 1.
20. Cohen-Solal.
21. Glueck.
22. Ibid.
23. Ibid.
24. Sheets.
25. Ibid.
26. Ibid.
27. Ibid.
28. Cooke.
29. Glueck.
30. Cooke.
31. Christopher Rothko, "Introduction" in *The Artist's Reality* by Mark Rothko (New Haven, CT: Yale Univ. Press, 2004), xi-xxxii.
32. Breslin, 532.
33. Ibid., 530.
34. Ibid.
35. Ibid.
36. Ibid.
37. Ibid.
38. Ibid.
39. Fisun Güner, "How Rothko Become the Mythic Superman of Mystical Abstraction," November 2014, https://www.spectator.co.uk/article/how-rothko-become-the-mythic-superman-of-mystical-abstraction.
40. Cooke.
41. Chave, 90.
42. Jacob Baal-Teshuva and Mark Rothko, *Rothko* (Köln: Taschen, 2015), 33.

JACOB LAWRENCE

1. Regenia A. Perry, "Free within Ourselves: African American Artists in the Collection of the National Museum of American Art," Smithsonian American Art Museum, accessed December 14, 2020, https://americanart.si.edu/artist/jacob-lawrence-2828.
2. "Jacob Lawrence: Painter of Black History and Life," MoMA, accessed December 14, 2020, https://www.moma.org/learn/moma_learning/jacob-lawrence-migration-series-1940-41/.
3. Perry.
4. Stephanie Dickinson, *Jacob Lawrence: Painter* (New York: Cavendish Square, 2017), 54.
5. Ibid.
6. "Keith Haring | Jean-Michel Basquiat: Crossing Lines," Transcript of Multimedia Guide, narrated by Patti Astor. (Victoria: National Gallery of Victoria, 2019).
7. Patricia Hills and Jacob Lawrence, *Painting Harlem Modern: The Art of Jacob Lawrence* (Berkeley, CA: University of California Press, 2019), 214.
8. Dickinson, 56.
9. Ibid.
10. John Duggleby, *Story Painter: the Life of Jacob Lawrence* (San Francisco, CA: Chronicle Books, 1998), 39.
11. Morgan Hampton, "Sedation [Jacob Lawrence]," Sartle, October 10, 2020, https://www.sartle.com/artwork/sedation-jacob-lawrence.
12. Dickinson, 56.

DIANE ARBUS

1. Jessie Wender, "The Subject of an Arbus," *New Yorker*, April 8, 2014, https://www.newyorker.com/culture/photobooth/the-subject-of-an-arbus.
2. Sean O'Hagan, "Diane Arbus: Portrait of a Photographer Review—a Disturbing Study," *Guardian* (Guardian News and Media, October 25, 2016), https://www.theguardian.com/books/2016/oct/25/diane-arbus-portrait-of-a-photographer-review-arthur-lubow.
3. William Todd Schultz, *An Emergency in Slow Motion: The Inner Life of Diane Arbus* (New York: Bloomsbury, 2013).
4. Jenna Ross, "Diane Arbus: Purveyor Photographer of the Weird and Wacky," TheCollector, April 28, 2020, https://www.thecollector.com/diane-arbus-photographer/.
5. Sigmund Freud, *Beyond the Pleasure Principle* (London: The International Psycho-Analytical Press, 1922), 79.
6. Anthony Bannon, "The Biography Diane Arbus Always Deserved," *Buffalo News*, June 26, 2016, https://buffalonews.com/lifestyles/the-biography-diane-arbus-alwaysdeserved/article_66f04335-f7a1-5e75-a039-9c2b6ebcb5ee.html.
7. Alex Mar, "The Cost of Diane Arbus's Life on the Edge," The Cut, July 12, 2016, https://www.thecut.com/2016/07/diane-arbus-c-v-r.html.
8. Diane Leach, "Diane Arbus: 'Happiness Perplexed Her,'" PopMatters, February 21, 2020, https://www.popmatters.com/diane-arbus-

portrait-of-a-photographer-by-arthurlubow-2495417010.html.

9. Deborah Nelson, *Tough Enough: Arbus, Arendt, Didion, McCarthy, Sontag, Weil* (Chicago, IL: University of Chicago Press, 2017), 121-122.
10. Lyle Rexler, "Through Her Lens Darkly: Diane Arbus's Life Was as Raw as Her Work," *New York Times*, July 1, 2016, https://www.nytimes.com/2016/07/03/books/review/diane-arbus-biography-by-arthur-lubow.html.
11. Parul Sehgal, "Diane Arbus's Sexual Adventures," BookForum, 2017.
12. Arthur Lubow, "The Woman Who Influenced Diane Arbus's Eye," *Wall Street Journal* (Dow Jones & Company, May 25, 2016) https://www.wsj.com/articles/the-woman-who-influenced-diane-arbuss-eye-1464187560.
13. Arthur Lubow and Diane Arbus, *Diane Arbus: Portrait of a Photographer* (New York, United States, NY: Ecco, an imprint of Harper Collins Publishers, 2017), 18-19.
14. Mar, "The Cost."
15. O'Hagan; and Ross.
16. O'Hagan.
17. Tara Murtha, "'Diane Arbus': Genius? Predator? Is There a Difference?," *Philadelphia Inquirer*, September 4, 2016, https://www.inquirer.com/philly/entertainment/20160904_Diane_Arbus_Genius_Predator_Is_there_a_difference_.html.
18. Leach.
19. Ross.
20. Jacqui Palumbo, "Revisiting Diane Arbus's Final and Most Contro versial Series," Artsy, November 8, 2018, https://www.artsy.net/article/artsy-editorial-revisiting-diane-arbuss-final-controversial-series.
21. *Masters of Photography: Diane Arbus* (Creative Arts Television Archive, Contemporary Arts Media (distributor), 1972).
22. Lane.
23. Bosworth, 269.

III. PROCESSING PAIN THROUGH ART: TRAUMA & PTSD

1. Elaine Mayers Salkaln, "The Mystery Woman," *New York Times Magazine*, October 3, 2002, p. 46.
2. Ann Hoff, "'I Was Convulsed, Pitiably Hideous': Convulsive Shock Treatment in Leonora Carrington's Down Below," *Journal of Modern Literature* 32, no. 3 (2009): pp. 83-98, https://doi.org/10.2979/jml.2009.32.3.83, 88.

GUSTAVE DORÉ

1. Blanche Roosevelt, *Life and Reminiscences of Gustave Dore´* (London: Sampson, 1885), 444.
2. Patricia Czapp and Kevin Kovach, "American Academy of Family Physicians," American Academy of Family Physicians, 2015, https://www.aafp.org/about/policies/all/poverty-health.html.
3. Blanchard Jerrold, "London: a Pilgrimage," in *London: a Pilgrimage* (Norwalk, CT: Easton Press, 2011), xvii.
4. Linda Nochlin, *Misère: The Visual Representation of Misery in the 19th Century* (London: Thames and Hudson, 2018). Ebook.
5. Roosevelt, 225.
6. Ibid.
7. Frank H. Norton, *Paul Gustave Dore´* (New York: J.B. Alden, 1883), 121.
8. "The Galaxy," United States: W.C. and F.P. Church, 1874, 351.
9. Maria Popova, "Gustave Doré's Hauntingly Beautiful 1883 Illustrations for Edgar Allan Poe's 'The Raven,'" Brain Pickings, January 19, 2016, https://www.brainpickings.org/2015/08/05/gustav-dore-poe-the-raven/.

FRIDA KAHLO

1. Gerry Souter, *Frida Kahlo: Beneath the Mirror* (New York: Parkstone, 2005), 201.
2. Salomon Grimberg, *Frida Kahlo: Song of Herself* (London: Merrell, 2008), 123.
3. Ibid., 19.
4. Ibid., 149.
5. R. Chris Fraley, "A Brief Overview of Adult Attachment Theory and Research," Department of Psychology University of Illinois at Urbana-Champaign, 2018, http://labs.psychology.illinois.edu/~rcfraley/attachment.htm.
6. Grimberg, 21.
7. Carol A. Courtney, Michael A. O'Hearn, and Carla C. Franck, "Frida Kahlo: Portrait of Chronic Pain," *Physical Therapy* 97, no. 1 (January 2017): pp. 90-96, https://doi.org/https://doi.org/10.2522/ptj.20160036.
8. Grimberg, 21
9. Gerardo Ochoa, "Museo Frida Kahlo," Museo Frida Kahlo, June 2020, https://www.museofridakahlo.org.mx/wp-content/uploads/2020/06/Frida_Kahlo_Bio-Gerardo_Ochoa-en.pdf, 3.
10. Grimberg, 23.
11. Daniel Bullen, *The Love Lives of the Artists: Five Stories of Creative Intimacy* (Berkeley, CA: Counterpoint Press, 2011), 190.
12. Hayden Herrera, foreword to *Frida Kahlo: Song of Herself*, by Salomon Grimberg (London: Merrell, 2008), 11.
13. Bullen, 177.
14. Celia Stahr, *Frida in America: the Creative Awakening of a Great Artist* (New York: St. Martin's Press, 2020).
15. Grimberg,100.

16. Stahr.
17. Mariana Medina and Sara McIntosh Wooten, *Frida Kahlo: Self-Portrait Artist* (New York: Enslow Publishing, 2016), 73.
18. Fernando Antelo, "Pain and the Paintbrush: The Life and Art of Frida Kahlo," *Virtual Mentor: American Medical Association Journal of Ethics* 15, no. 5 (May 2013): pp. 460-465, https://journalofethics.ama-assn.org/article/painand-paintbrush-life-and-art-frida-kahlo/2013-05, 462.
19. Grimberg, 22.
20. Ibid., 129.
21. Antelo, 462.
22. Grimberg, 118.
23. Ibid., 118-119.
24. Lupe Rocha, "Kahlo's Reflection: The Absence of Equal Ability," Medium, July 27, 2018, https://medium.com/@luperoach/kahlos-reflection-the-absence-of-equal-ability-4e5d88504f9a.
25. Ibid.
26. Grimberg, 128.
27. Frida Kahlo, "I'm Amputating You," Letters of Note, July 6, 2020, https://lettersofnote.com/2020/07/06/im-amputating-you/.
28. Grimberg, 127.
29. Antelo, 461.
30. Ibid., 463

LEONORA CARRINGTON

1. Anwen Crawford, "Leonora Carrington Rewrote the Surrealist Narrative for Women," 2017, https://www.newyorker.com/books/page-turner/leonora-carrington-rewrote-the-surrealist-narrative-for-women.
2. Marina Warner, "Introduction" in *Down Below* by Leonora Carrington. (New York: New York Review of Books, 2017), p. vii-xxxiv.
3. Lauren Butterworth, "Leonora Carrington," Deviant Women, podcast audio, March 15, 2017 https://deviantwomenpodcast.com/2017/03/16/leonora-carrington/.
4. Ibid.; and Elaine Mayers Salkaln, "The Mystery Woman," *New York Times*, October 13, 2002, https://www.nytimes.com/2002/10/13/magazine/the-mysterywoman.html, 50; and Roberta Smith, "Female Surrealists Re-Emerge in 2 Startling Shows," *New York Times*, 2019, https://www.nytimes.com/2019/06/13/arts/design/leonora-carrington-paintings.html.
5. Warner.
6. Leonora Carrington, "The Debutante," in *The Complete Stories of Leonora Carrington* (St. Louis, MO: Dorothy Project, 2017).
7. Ibid.
8. Butterworth
9. Ibid.
10. Susannah Rigg, "Leonora Carrington Museum Is a Surreal Location for Surrealist Art," July 10, 2018, https://mexiconewsdaily.com/mexicolife/leonora-carrington-museum/.

11. Ibid.
12. Ibid.
13. Leonora Carrington, "Monday, 23 August 1943," in *Down Below* (New York: New York Review of Books, 2017), https://www.europenow journal.org/2017/01/04/down-below-by-leonora-carrington/.
14. Justin Goodman, "Down Below, a Memoir by Leonora Carrington, Reviewed," Cleaver Magazine (Cleaver Magazine, June 18, 2020), https://www.cleavermagazine.com/down-below-a-memoir-by-leonora-carrington-reviewed-byjustin-goodman/.
15. Crawford.
16. Butterworth
17. Crawford.
18. Carrington, "Monday."
19. Ibid.
20. Carrington, "Monday."
21. Crawford.
22. Carrington, "Monday."
23. Warner.
24. Ibid.
25. Crawford.
26. Ann Hoff, "'I Was Convulsed, Pitiably Hideous': Convulsive Shock Treatment in Leonora Carrington's Down Below," *Journal of Modern Literature* 32, no. 3 (2009): pp. 83-98, https://doi.org/10.2979/jml.2009.32.3.83, 83.
27. Hoff, 83.
28. Hoff, 83.
29. Elisa Wouk Almino, "The Idiosyncratic Writings of Leonora Carrington, a Reluctant Surrealist," Hyperallergic, June 20, 2017, https://hyperallergic.com/374789/the-idiosyncratic-writings-of-leonora-carrington-a-reluctantsurrealist/.
30. Hoff, 88
31. Walsh.
32. Sehgal.
33. Walsh.
34. James Hewison and Michelle Man, *Leonora Carrington: Living Legacies* (Wilmington, DE: Vernon Press, 2020), 95.
35. Crawford.
36. Almino.
37. Warner.
38. Ibid.
39. Sehgal.
40. Laity; and Sehgal.
41. Warner.
42. Salkaln.
43. Walsh.

BODY IMAGE AND ART

1. Subhashini Ganesan, SL Ravishankar, and Sudha Ramalingam, "Are Body Image Issues Affecting Our Adolescents? A Cross-Sectional Study among College Going Adolescent Girls," *Indian Journal of Community Medicine* 43, no. 5 (2018): p. 42, https://doi.org/10.4103/ijcm.ijcm_62_18.
2. Sotheby's, "Jenny Saville and the Beauty of Individualism," Sothebys.com (Sotheby's, February 18, 2019), https://www.sothebys.com/en/articles/jenny-saville-and-the-beauty-of-individualism.

YAYOI KUSAMA

1. Yayoi Kusama and Ralph F. McCarthy, *Infinity Net: The Autobiography of Yayoi Kusama* (London: Tate, 2020).
2. Justin McCurry, "Justin McCurry Talks to Artist Yayoi Kusama," *Guardian* (Guardian News and Media, June 5, 2009), https://www.theguardian.com/artanddesign/2009/jun/06/yayoi-kusama-art.
3. *Kusama: Infinity*, Hulu, 2018, https://www.hulu.com/movie/kusama-infinity-b3d0bfc5-3b1e-4132-808f-91da354fdde0.
4. Ibid.
5. *Kusama: Infinity*, 2018
6. Ibid.
7. Ibid.
8. James Romaine, "Yayoi Kusama's Infinity Nets: Sublime or Spectacle?," Comment Magazine, June 5, 2009, https://www.cardus.ca/comment/article/yayoi-kusamas-infinity-nets-sublime-or-spectacle/.
9. Applin, 4.
10. *Kusama: Infinity*, 2018.
11. Kusama, "Autobiography."
12. Kusama, "Autobiography."
13. Ibid.
14. *Self-Obliteration* (Shady Film Productions, 1967).
15. Kusama, "Autobiography."
16. Helen Holmes, "Yayoi Kusama Just Published a Poem About the 'Terrible Monster' Coronavirus," *Observer* (Observer, April 15, 2020), https://observer.com/2020/04/yayoi-kusama-poetry-coronavirus/.
17. *Kusama: Infinity*, 2018

INSTITUTIONAL RACISM AND TRAUMA

1. "The Body Remembers," Heather Agyepong, Multidisciplinary Artist/Actor, 2021, http://www.heatheragyepong.com/the-body-remembers.
2. Christabel Johanson, "Mental Health in Black Art," Africanah.org. September 7, 2020, https://africanah.org/mental-health-in-black-art/.
3. Jasmine Weber, "A Portrait of Black Mental Health in Hues of Black

and Blue," Hyperallergic, July 12, 2019, https://hyperallergic.com/469609/a-portrait-of-black-mental-health-in-hues-of-black-and-blue/.

JEAN-MICHEL BASQUIAT

1. Cathleen McGuigan, "New Art, New Money," *New York Times Magazine*, 1985, sec. 6, p. 20, https://www.nytimes.com/1985/02/10/magazine/new-art-new-money.html.
2. Anthony Haden-Guest, "Burning Out," Vanity Fair, November 1988, https://www.vanityfair.com/news/1988/11/jean-michel-basquiat.
3. "Dual Diagnosis," National Alliance on Mental Illness, March 2015, https://www.nami.org/NAMI/media/NAMIMedia/Images/Fact Sheets/Dual-Diagnosis-FS.pdf.
4. Davis, Tamra, dir. *Jean-Michel Basquiat: The Radiant Child*. DVD. USA: Arthouse Films, 2011.
5. Phoebe Hoban, *Basquiat: A Quick Killing in Art* (New York: Viking, 1998).
6. Aisha Sabatini Sloan, "On Basquiat, the Black Body, and a Strange Sensation in My Neck," Paris Review, October 26, 2017, https://www.theparisreview.org/blog/2017/10/26/basquiat-black-body-strange-sensation-neck/.
7. Hoban, Basquiat: A Quick Killing in Art.
8. Ibid.
9. Ibid.
10. Ibid.
11. Tori DeAngelis, "The Legacy of Trauma," *Monitor on Psychology* 50, no. 2 (February 2019): p. 36, https://www.apa.org/monitor/2019/02/legacy-trauma.
12. Ibid.
13. Ibid.
14. Ibid.
15. Hoban, *Basquiat: A Quick Killing in Art.*
16. Ibid.
17. Nikitta Foston, "Behind the Pain Nobody Talks About: Sexual Abuse of Black Boy," *Ebony*, June 2003.
18. McGuigan.
19. Hoban, *Basquiat: A Quick Killing in Art.*
20. Constance L. Hays, "Jean Basquiat, 27, An Artist of Words and Angular Images," *New York Times*, 1988, sec. D, p. 11, https://www.nytimes.com/1988/08/15/obituaries/jeanbasquiat-27-an-artist-of-words-and-angular-images.html.
21. Raynor.
22. *Jean-Michel Basquiat: The Radiant Child.*
23. Ibid.
24. Michael Wines, "Jean Michel Basquiat: Hazards of Sudden Success and Fame," *New York Times*, 1988, sec. 1, p. 9, https://www.nytimes.com/1988/08/27/arts/jean-michelbasquiat-hazards-of-sudden-success-and-fame.html.
25. Haden-Guest.

26. Wines.
27. Ibid.
28. *Jean-Michel Basquiat: The Radiant Child.*
29. Peter Schjeldahl, "Basquiat's Memorial to a Young Artist Killed By Police," *The New Yorker*, July 2019, https://www. newyorker.com/ magazine/2019/07/08/basquiats-memorial-to-a-young-artist -killed-by-police.
30. *Jean-Michel Basquiat: The Radiant Child.*
31. Ibid.
32. Schjeldahl.
33. *Jean-Michel Basquiat: The Radiant Child.*
34. Ibid.
35. Haden-Guest.
36. Ally Faughnan, "The Best, Worst, and Weirdest Parts of Warhol and Basquiat's Friendship," Dazed, May 28, 2019, https://www.dazed digital.com/art-photography/article/44600/1/never-before-seen -photos-diary-andy-warhol-jean-michelbasquiat-friendship.
37. Wines.
38. Haden-Guest.
39. Ibid.
40. Ibid.

GENDER IDENTITY AND DYSPHORIA

1. Cecilia Dhejne et al., "Mental Health and Gender Dysphoria: A Review of the Literature," *International Review of Psychiatry* 28, no. 1 (February 2016): pp. 44-57, https://doi.org/10.3109/09540261.2015. 1115753.
2. Joseph B. Treaster, "Overlooked No More: Claude Cahun, Whose Photographs Explored Gender and Sexuality," *New York Times*, June 19, 2019. https://www.nytimes.com/2019/06/19/obituaries/claude-cahun-overlooked.html

IV. DIFFERENT WAYS OF SEEING: SCHIZOPHRENIA AND OUTSIDER ART

1. Wendy Steiner, "In Love With the Myth of the 'Outsider'," New York Times, March 10, 1996, p. 45, https://www. nytimes.com/1996/03 /10/arts/art-view-in-love-with-themyth-of-the-outsider.html.
2. Linda Rainaldi, 2015, "Outsider Art : Forty Years Out," p. 2, Electronic Theses and Dissertations (ETDs) 2008+. T, University of British Columbia. doi:http://dx.doi.org/10.14288/1.0221495.
3. Ibid., 10.
4. Steiner.
5. Rainaldi, 54.
6. Clayton Schuster, "In NYC, a Fair Dedicated to Outsider Art Cultivates an Interest in the Eccentric," *Observer*, 2020, https://observer.com/

2020/01/outsider-art-fair-market-growth-in-new-york/.
7. Steiner.
8. Jenna Ross, "Diane Arbus: Purveyor Photographer of the Weird and Wacky," TheCollector, April 28, 2020, https://www.thecollector.com/diane-arbus-photographer/.
9. Rainaldi, 20.

RICHARD DADD

1. William Wood, *Remarks On the Plea of Insanity, and On the Management of Criminal Lunatics* (London: Longman, Brown, Green, and Longmans, 1851), 41.
2. David Bell, "Richard Dadd," Living With Schizophrenia, September 30, 2019, https://livingwithschizophreniauk.org/richard-dadd/.
3. Ibid.
4. Michael Prodger, "The Dangerous Mind of Richard Dadd," NewStatesman, July 2, 2015, https://www.newstatesman.com/culture/2015/07/dangerous-mind-richard-dadd.
5. Bell.
6. JMS Pearce, "Richard Dadd: Art and Madness," *Hektoen International* 11, no. 4 (2019).
7. Bell.
8. Ibid.
9. Prodger.
10. Bell.
11. Allan Beveridge, "Richard Dadd: The Artist and the Asylum, By Nicholas Tromans," *British Journal of Psychiatry* 200, no. 4 (2012): 349-50. doi:10.1192/bjp.bp.111.105957.
12. Bell.
13. Ibid.
14. Ibid.
15. Ibid.
16. Terry Trainor, *Bedlam: St. Mary of Bethlehem*, (self-pub., Lulu.com, 2010).
17. Andrew Scull, Charlotte MacKenzie, and Nicholas Hervey, *Masters of Bedlam: The Transformation of the Mad-Doctoring Trade* (Princeton, NJ: Princeton University Press, 2014), 3.
18. Ibid., 11.
19. Bell.
20. Charles A. Sarnoff, *Symbols in Structure and Function*, vol. 3 (Xlibris Corp., 2003), 222.
21. Prodger.
22. Frances Fowle, "'The Fairy Feller's Master-Stroke', Richard Dadd, 1855-64," Tate, 2000, https://www.tate.org.uk/art/artworks/dadd-the-fairy-fellers-master-stroke-t00598.
23. Prodger.
24. Fowle.
25. Nicholas Tromans, "Richard Dadd: The Artist and the Asylum—TateShots," Tate, February 9, 2012, https://www. tate.org.uk/art/

artists/richard-dadd-130/richard-dadd-artist-and-asylum.

26. Bell.
27. *A Handbook to the Water Colours, Drawings, and Engravings in the Art Treasures Exhibition: Being a Reprint of Critical Notices Originally Published in "The Manchester Guardian."* (London: Bradbury and Evans, 1857), 14.
28. Carolina Irving, Miguel Flores-vianna, and Charlotte Di Carcaci, "Bohemian Rhapsody," *New York Times* (New York Times, February 10, 2015), https://www.nytimes.com/2015/02/10/t-magazine/in-the-air-bohemian-rhapsody.html.
29. A. S. Byatt, "Richard Dadd: the Fairy King," *Guardian* (Guardian News and Media, September 2, 2011), https://www.theguardian.com/artanddesign/2011/sep/02/richarddadd-fairy-king-byatt; and Neil Gaiman, "The Fairy Feller's Master Stroke," Neil Gaiman's Journal: The Fairy Feller's Master Stroke, January 1, 1970, http://journal.neilgaiman.com/2008/04/fairy-fellers-master-stroke.html.
30. Tate, "'The Flight out of Egypt', Richard Dadd, 1849-50," Tate, accessed January 4, 2021, https://www.tate.org.uk/art/artworks/dadd-the-flight-out-of-egypt-n05767.
31. Prodger.
32. Rudolf Arnheim, "The Art of Psychotics," *Art Psychotherapy* 4, no. 3-4 (1977): pp. 113-120, https://doi.org/10.1016/0090-9092(77)90026-6, 116.
33. Trainor.
34. Prodger.
35. Ibid,14.
36. Scull, 123-160.
37. Ibid.
38. Alexander Morison, *The Blackhalls of That Ilk and Barra, Hereditary Coronies and Foresters of the Garioch* (Aberdeen, Scotland: New Spalding Club, 1905), 115.
39. Jacqueline Banerjee, "Sir Alexander Morison by Richard Dadd, 1817-1886," VictorianWeb, June 27, 2020, http://www.victorianweb.org/painting/dadd/paintings/7.html.
40. Bell.
41. Trainor.
42. Trainor.
43. Tromans.
44. "The Anti-Psychiatry Movement," Living With Schizophrenia, September 19, 2017, https://livingwithschizophreniauk.org/information-sheets/the-anti-psychiatry-movement/.
45. Davidson, 1074.
46. Ibid.

LOUIS WAIN

1. Dale, Rodney. *Louis Wain: The Man Who Drew Cats*. London: Kimber, 1968, 2.
2. Heidi J. Wehring and William T. Carpenter, "Violence and Schizophrenia," Schizophrenia bulletin (Oxford University Press, September 2011), https://www.ncbi.nlm.nih.gov/pmc/articles/PMC3160236/.
3. Ibid.
4. Joseph Milton, "How a Mental Disorder Opened up an Invisible World of Colour and Pattern," Scientific American Blog Network (Scientific American, December 22, 2011), https://blogs.scientificamerican.com/creatology/how-a-mental-disorder-opened-up-an-invisible-world-of-colour-and-pattern/.
5. Paul Gallagher, "The Psychedelic Madness of Louis Wain's Cats," DangerousMinds, May 29, 2016, https://dangerousm inds.net/comments/the_psychedelic_madness_of_louis_wains_cats.
6. Paul Sorene, "Louis Wain: The Man Who Drew Millions of Far-Out Cats," Flashbak, July 3, 2018, https://flashbak.com/louis-wain-cats-403104/.
7. Chris Philo, "Royal College of Physicians of Edinburgh," Royal College of Physicians of Edinburgh (November 20, 2019).
8. Sorene.
9. Paul Moody, "The Forgotten Artist Who Changed the Way We Look at Cats," AnotherMan, October 18, 2018, https://www.anothermanmag.com/life-culture/10560/the-forgotten-artist-who-changed-the-way-we-look-at-catslouis-wain.
10. Milton.
11. Sidney Denham, "The Man Who Drew Cats: From the Archive, 5 August 1960," *Guardian* (Guardian News and Media, August 5, 2013), https://www.theguardian.com/theguardian/2013/aug/05/cats-louis-wain-illustrations.
12. Milton.
13. Philo, 15:33.
14. Ransom Riggs, "Did Cats Drive This Painter Insane?," Mental Floss, November 9, 2010, https://www.mentalfloss.com/article/26328/did-cats-drive-painter-insane.
15. Philo, 20:30.
16. Philip Kennedy, "Cute Cats and Psychedelia: The Tragic Life of Louis Wain," Illustration Chronicles, November 2016, https://illustrationchronicles.com/Cute-Cats-and-Psychedelia-The-Tragic-Life-of-Louis-Wain.
17. Ibid.
18. Philo, 4:32.
19. Ibid., 20:30.
20. Ibid., 10:12.
21. Ibid., 10:54.
22. Moody.
23. Philo, 12:35.
24. Ibid,14:08.
25. David O'Flynn, "Bethlem Museum of the Mind," Bethlem Museum of

the Mind (2012), https://www.youtube.com/watch?v=KTwbTgX_imE, 4:21

26. Silvia Helena Cardoso, "Cats Painted in the Progression of Psychosis of a Schizophrenic Artist," Neuroscience Art Gallery, accessed September 21, 2020, https://cerebromente.org.br/gallery/gall_leonardo/fig1-a.htm.
27. Milton.
28. Gallagher.
29. Sorene.
30. Moody.
31. "The Curious Cats of Louis Wain," YouTube, 2018.
32. Danielle Watson, "Psychotic Diagnosis and Artist Pathology: Schizophrenic Art's Influence on the Identification of the Disorder" (2014), Honors Projects, 7. https://scholarworks.bgsu.edu/honorsprojects/160
33. Ibid., 3.
34. Ibid., 11.

ALOÏSE CORBAZ

1. Jina Valentine, *Ticket to the Unknown* (United States: Future Plan and Program, 2011), 37.
2. B.S. Ruoss, *The Subject of Schizophrenia—All You Want To Know About the Illness* (Xlibris US, 2020).
3. Charles Russell, "Aloïse Corbaz," Outsider Art Fair, accessed November 18, 2020, https://www.outsiderartfair.com/artists/aloise-corbaz.
4. Ibid.
5. Danilo Campanella, *New Horizons: Europe's Death and the Birth of a New World*, trans. Giada Ferioli (Italy: Youcanprint, 2019).
6. Ibid.
7. Céline Muzelle, "The Art of Aloïse: A Lone Continent?," Raw Vision, 2012, https://rawvision.com/articles/art-aloise-lone-continent.
8. Russell.
9. "Aloïse Corbaz 1886-1964," Raw Vision, accessed November 18, 2020, https://rawvision.com/sourcebook/aloise-corbaz-1886-1964.
10. Muzelle.
11. Michele Laird, "The Creative Schizophrenia of Aloïse," swissinfo.ch (swissinfo.ch, November 6, 2017), https://www.swissinfo.ch/eng/drugs-and-creativity_the-creative-schizophrenia-of-aloise/33250538.
12. Valentine, 10.
13. Ibid., 13.
14. Ibid., 14.
15. Ruoss.
16. "Aloïse Corbaz 1886-1964"
17. Jacqueline Porret-Forel, "Aloïse & the Theater of the Universe," accessed November 18, 2020, https://ubu.com/ethno/visuals/aloise.html.

18. Ibid.
19. Ibid.
20. "The Art Brut of Aloïse Corbaz," Schiz Life, January 12, 2016, http://www.schizlife.com/the-art-brut-of-aloise-corbaz/.
21. Muzelle.
22. Laird.

AGNES MARTIN

1. Agnes Martin, *Writings*, ed. Dieter Schwarz (Ostfildern: Edition Cantz, 1993), 16.
2. Miranda.
3. Holland Cotter, "The Joy of Reading Between Agnes Martin's Lines," *New York Times*, 2016, sec. C, p. 21, https://www.nytimes.com/2016/10/07/arts/design/the-joy-of-readingbetween-agnes-martins-lines.html.
4. Hilton Als, "The Heroic Art of Agnes Martin," *New York Review of Books*, July 14, 2016.
5. Ibid.
6. Ibid.
7. "Agnes Martin," Pace Gallery, accessed November 18, 2020, https://www.pacegallery.com/artists/agnes-martin/.
8. Cotter.
9. Ibid.
10. Carolina A. Miranda, "Q&A: What the World Misunderstands about Artist Agnes Martin and How Her Biographer Unearthed Her Story," *Los Angeles Times*, 2016, https://www. latimes.com/entertainment/arts/miranda/la-et-cam-agnesmartin-nancy-princenthal-biography-lacma-20160411-column.html.
11. Olivia Laing, "Agnes Martin: the Artist Mystic Who Disappeared into the Desert," *Guardian*, 2015, https://www.theguardian.com/artanddesign/2015/may/22/agnesmartin-the-artist-mystic-who-disappeared-into-the-desert; and Henry Martin, *Agnes Martin: Pioneer, Painter, Icon* (Tucson, AZ: Schaffner Press, Inc, 2018).
12. Henry Martin, *Agnes Martin: Pioneer, Painter, Icon* (Tucson, AZ: Schaffner Press, Inc, 2018).
13. Miranda; and Jennifer Harris, "Agnes Martin: MoMA," The Museum of Modern Art, 2016, https://www.moma.org/artists/3787.
14. Cotter.
15. Miranda.
16. Cotter.
17. John Gruen, "Agnes Martin: 'Everything, Everything Is about Feeling…Feeling and Recognition'," ARTnews, 1976, https://www.artnews.com/art-news/retrospective/what-we-make-is-what-we-feel-agnes-martin-on-hermeditative-practice-in-1976-4630/.
18. Ibid.
19. Ibid.
20. Nancy Princenthal, *Agnes Martin: Her Life and Art* (London: Thames and Hudson, 2015), 124.

21. https://www.sfaq.us/2016/08/the-poetics-of-the-grid-agnes-martin-at-lacma/
22. Martin, 29.
23. https://www.sfaq.us/2016/08/the-poetics-of-the-grid-agnes-martin-at-lacma/
24. Laing.
25. Princenthal, 120.
26. Ibid.
27. Miranda.
28. Gruen.

BIBLIOGRAPHY

VINCENT VAN GOGH

Bailey, Martin. *Starry Night: Van Gogh at the Asylum*. London: White Lion, 2018.

Bhattacharyya, Kalyan B., and Saurabh Rai. "The Neuropsychiatric Ailment of Vincent Van Gogh." *Annals of Indian Academy of Neurology* 18, no. 1 (2015): 6-9.

Blumer, Dietrich. "The Illness of Vincent Van Gogh." *American Journal of Psychiatry* 159, no. 4 (April 2002): 519-26.

Cascone, Sarah. "Doctors Cannot Figure Out Vincent Van Gogh's Illness." Artnet News, September 17, 2016.

Dietrich, Arne. "The Mythconception of the Mad Genius." *Frontiers in Psychology*, February 2014.

Gogh, Vincent van. *Ever Yours: The Essential Letters*. Edited by Leo Jansen, Hans Luijten, and Nienke Bakker. New Haven, CT: Yale University Press, 2014.

Jones, Jonathan. "Vincent Van Gogh: Myths, Madness and a New Way of Painting." *Guardian*, August 5, 2016.

Popova, Maria. "Van Gogh and Mental Illness." *Brain Pickings*, March 30, 2017.

Simonton, Dean Keith. "Are Genius and Madness Related? Contemporary Answers to an Ancient Question." *Psychiatric Times* 22, no. 7 (May 2005).

"Vincent Van Gogh Quotes (Author of *The Letters of Vincent Van Gogh*)." Goodreads.com.

Williams, Katherine. *Women on the Verge: The Culture of Neurasthenia in Nineteenth-Century America*. Stanford, CA: Iris & B. Gerald Cantor Center for Visual Arts at Stanford University, 2004.

Wright, Craig. "Is There a Thin Line between Genius and Insanity?" *Psychology Today*, 2020.

MICHELANGELO BUONARROTI

"Any Mood Disorder." National Institute of Mental Health, US Department of Health and Human Services, 2017. nimh.nih.gov.

Crompton, Louis. *Homosexuality & Civilization*. Cambridge, MA: Belknap Press of Harvard University Press, 2006.

Gayford, Martin. *Michelangelo: His Epic Life*. London: Penguin UK, 2013.

King, Ross. *Michelangelo & the Pope's Ceiling*. London: Penguin Books, 2003.

Kristof, Jane. "Michelangelo as Nicodemus: The Florence Pieta." *Sixteenth Century Journal* 20, no. 2 (1989): 163-82.

Kromm, Jane. "Psychological States and the Artist: The Problem of Michelangelo." *Studies in Visual Communication* 6, no. 1 (1980): 69-76.

Lewis, J. Patrick, and Michelangelo Buonarroti. *Michelangelo's World*. Mankato, MN: Creative Editions, 2007.

Michelangelo. *Complete Poems of Michelangelo*. Translated by John Frederick Nims. Chicago: University of Chicago Press, 2000.

Nims, John Frederick. Preface. In *Complete Poems of Michelangelo*, xvii-xxi. Chicago: University of Chicago Press, 2000.

Pope-Hennessy, John Wyndham. *An Introduction to Italian Sculpture: Italian High Renaissance and Baroque Sculpture*. London: Phaidon, 1963.

Saslow, James M. "James M. Saslow on Sensuality and Spirituality in Michelangelo's Poetry." metmuseum.org, 2018.

Somervill, Barbara A. *Michelangelo: Sculptor and Painter*. Minneapolis: Capstone, 2008.

Stone, Irving. "'Improbable' Story of 'The Pieta.'" *New York Times*, April 22, 1962, sec. SM.

Storr, Anthony. *Solitude: A Return to the Self*. New York: Simon and Schuster, 2005.

Ziegler, Joanna E. "Michelangelo and the Medieval Pietà: The Sculpture of Devotion or the Art of Sculpture?" *Gesta* 34, no. 1 (1995): 28-36.

FRANCISCO GOYA

Casey, Laura L. "Goya: 'In Sickness and in Health.'" *International Journal of Surgery* 4, no. 1 (2006).

Chang, Larry. *Wisdom for the Soul: Five Millennia of Prescriptions for Spiritual Healing*. Washington, DC: Gnosophia Publishers, 2006.

Felisati, D., and G. Sperati. "Francisco Goya and His Illness." *Acta Otorhinolaryngologica Italica: Organo Ufficiale Della Società Italiana Di Otorinolaringologia e Chirurgia Cervico-Facciale* 30 (October 5, 2010): 264-270.

Henry, Alan E. H. "*The Madhouse* by Francisco Goya." *Practical Neurology* 3 (2003).

Hughes, Robert. *Goya*. New York: Knopf Doubleday Publishing Group, 2012.

Klein, Peter K. "Insanity and the Sublime: Aesthetics and Theories of Mental Illness in Goya's *Yard with Lunatics* and Related Works." *Journal of the Warburg and Courtauld Institutes* 61.

MacLean, Robert. "Los Caprichos." Glasgow University Library Special Collections Department, 2006.

Novotney, Amy. "The Risks of Social Isolation." *Monitor on Psychology* 50, no. 5 (2019).

Simonton, Dean Keith. "Are Genius and Madness Related? Contemporary Answers to an Ancient Question." *Psychiatric Times* 22, no. 7 (2005).

Toptan, Tugce, et al. "Neurosyphilis: a Case Report." *Northern Clinics of Istanbul* 2, no. 1 (2015).

Voorhies, James. "Francisco De Goya (1746-1828) and the Spanish Enlightenment." metmuseum.org, 2003.

DISABILITY AND ILLNESS

Sulewski, Jennifer Sullivan, Heike Boeltzig, and Rooshey Hasnain. "Art and Disability: Intersecting Identities among Young Artists with Disabilities." *Disability Studies Quarterly* 32, no. 1 (2012). https://doi.org/10.18061/dsq.v32i1.3034.

Turner, R. Jay, and Samuel Noh. "Physical Disability and Depression: A Longitudinal Analysis." *Journal of Health and Social Behavior* 29, no. 1 (1988): 23. https://doi.org/10.2307/2137178.

EDVARD MUNCH

Azeem, Hina. "The Art of Edvard Munch: A Window onto a Mind." *BJPsych Advances* 21, no. 1 (2015): 51-53.

Beams, Sophia. "*The Scream*: A Deeper Analysis of Edvard Munch's Anxiety-Wrought Piece." Medium. Everything Art, August 2, 2019.

Cascone, Sarah. "Doctors Cannot Figure Out Vincent Van Gogh's Illness." Artnet News, September 17, 2016.

Ebert, Andreas, and Karl-Jürgen Bär. "Emil Kraepelin: A Pioneer of Scientific Understanding of Psychiatry and Psychopharmacology." *Indian Journal of Psychiatry* 52, no. 2 (April 2010): 191-92.

Harris, James C. "Art and Images in Psychiatry." *Archives of General Psychiatry* 64, no. 9 (2007): 996-97.

Lubow, Arthur. "Edvard Munch: Beyond *The Scream*." *Smithsonian Magazine*, March 2006.

Maletic, Vladimir. "Differentiating between Bipolar and Schizoaffective Diagnoses." *Psychiatry & Behavioral Health Learning Network*, March 6, 2020.

Mann, Jon. "How Edvard Munch Expressed the Anxiety of the Modern World." *Artsy*, July 10, 2017.

Papolos, Demitri F., and Janice Papolos. *The Bipolar Child (Third Edition): The Definitive and Reassuring Guide to Childhood's Most Misunderstood Disorder*. New York: Broadway Books, 2006.

Preda, Adrian. "The Difference between Schizophrenia and Schizoaffective Disorder." Verywell Mind, January 31, 2020.

Prideaux, Sue. *Edvard Munch: Behind* The Scream. New Haven, CT: Yale University Press, 2019.

Rothenberg, Albert. "Bipolar Illness, Creativity, and Treatment." *Psychiatric Quarterly* 72, no. 2 (2001): 131-47.

Rothenberg, Albert. "Creativity and Mental Illness II: *The Scream*." *Psychology Today*. Sussex Publishers, March 24, 2015.

Warick, Lawrence, and Elaine Warick. "Edvard Munch: A Study of Loss, Grief and Creativity." msu.edu.

Yafi, Michael. " Edvard Munch: The Child Who Never Grew Up." Hektoen International, 2019.

INFLUENCE ON CONTEMPORARY ARTISTS: TRACEY EMIN

Higgie, Jennifer. "Tracey Emin's Lifelong Affinity with Edvard Munch." Royal Academy of Arts, November 30, 2020. https://www.royalacademy.org.uk/article/tracey-emin-jennifer-higgie-interview.

Waugh, Rosemary. "The Enduring Connection between Art and Mental Health." Art UK, November 4, 2020. https://artuk.org/discover/stories/the-enduring-connection-between-art-and-mental-health.

GEORGIA O'KEEFFE

Andrew, Jason. "A Painter's Retreat: Georgia O'Keeffe and Lake George." Hyperallergic, July 18, 2013.

"Anxiety Disorders." Mayo Clinic. Mayo Foundation for Medical Education and Research, May 4, 2018.

Boxer, Sarah. "Georgia O'Keeffe, That Crazy Little Girl." *New York Times*, August 1, 1997, sec. C.

Bullen, Daniel. *The Love Lives of the Artists: Five Stories of Creative Intimacy*. Berkeley, CA: Counterpoint, 2011.

Cotter, Holland. "World War I—The Quick. The Dead. The Artists." *New York Times*, January 6, 2017, sec. C.

Cuncic, Arlin. "What High Functioning Anxiety Feels Like." Verywell Mind, May 11, 2020.

Drohojowska-Philp, Hunter. *Full Bloom: The Art and Life of Georgia O'Keeffe*. New York: W. W. Norton, 2006.

"Facts & Statistics." Anxiety and Depression Association of America (ADAA).

Laing, Olivia. "The Wild Beauty of Georgia O'Keeffe." *Guardian*, July 1, 2016.

Messinger, Lisa. "Georgia O'Keeffe (1887-1986)." metmuseum.org, 2004.

O'Keeffe, Georgia, and Alfred Stieglitz. *My Faraway One: Selected Letters of Georgia O'Keeffe and Alfred Stieglitz*. Edited by Sarah Greenough. New Haven, CT: Yale University Press, 2011.

O'Keeffe, Georgia, and Amy Von Lintel. *Georgia O'Keeffe's Wartime Texas Letters*. College Station: Texas A&M University Press, 2020.

Popova, Maria. "Georgia O'Keeffe on Art, Life, and Setting Priorities." *Brain Pickings*, November 16, 2019.

Prypchan, Lida. "Georgia O'Keeffe (Part I)." Medium, October 15, 2020.

Robinson, Roxana. *Georgia O'Keeffe: A Life*. London: Bloomsbury, 2020.

Robinson, Roxana. "The Rivalry between Georgia O'Keeffe and Her Sister Ida." *New Yorker*, September 4, 2017.

Rose, Phyllis. *Alfred Stieglitz: Taking Pictures, Making Painters*. New Haven, CT: Yale University Press, 2019.

Scott, Nancy J. *Georgia O'Keeffe (Critical Lives)*. Durrington, UK: Reaktion Books (UK), 2015.

Udall, Sharyn R. "Georgia O'Keeffe and Emily Carr: Health, Nature and the Creative Process." *Women's Art Journal* 27, no. 1 (2006): 17-25.

JOAN MIRÓ

Bogousslavsky, Julien, and Laurent Tatu. *Neurological Disorders in Famous Artists*. Basel, Switzerland: Karger, 2018.

Canaday, John. "Calder and Miró: One's Mobiles, the Other's Paintings, in a Just About Perfect Show." *New York Times*, February 26, 1961, sec. X.

Delgado, Montserrat G., and Julien Bogousslavsky. "Joan Miró and Cyclic Depression." *Frontiers of Neurology and Neuroscience* 43 (2018): 1-7.

Gibson, Michael. "An Uneasy Stroll through Early Miró." *International Herald Tribune*, March 6, 2004.

Gonzalez, Mike. "Joan Miro: A Blow between the Eyes." *Socialist Review*, June 2011, 359.

Kimmelman, Michael. "The Creative Mind Reader." *New York Times*, December 31, 2006, National edition, sec. 6.

Meisler, Stanley. "For Joan Miró, Poetry and Painting Were the Same." *Smithsonian Magazine*, November 1993.

Mink, Janis, and Miró Joan. *Joan Miró 1893—1983*. Cologne: Taschen, 1993.

Miró, Joan. "Aidez L'Espagne [Help Spain]." National Galleries of Scotland. Accessed December 9, 2020.

Miró, Joan, Robert Lubar, and Yvon Taillandier. *Joan Miró: I Work Like a Gardener (Interview with Joan Miró on His Creative Process)*. Edited by Kevin C. Lippert. New York: Princeton Architectural Press, 2017.

Popova, Maria. "I Work Like a Gardener: Joan Miró on Art, Motionless Movement, and the Proper Pace of Creative Labor." *Brain Pickings*, September 18, 2018.

Reyburn, Scott. "Banksy and Rembrandt Boost Sotheby's Sale to $192.7 Million." *New York Times*, July 30, 2020.

Richardson, John. "Hidden Miró." *Vanity Fair*, September 1993.

Schildkraut, Joseph J. "Opinion: Miró Offers Case in Point of Creativity's Link to Depression." *New York Times*, October 24, 1993, sec. 4.

Thornton-Cronin, Lesley. "Unicorn Poop: Did a Surrealist Do It First?" Medium. VantagePoint: Visual Culture, September 18, 2020.

ALICE NEEL

Allara, Pamela, and Alice Neel. *Pictures of People: Alice Neel's American Portrait Gallery*. Waltham, MA: Brandeis University Press, 2000.

Bauer, Denise. "Alice Neel's Portraits of Mother Work." *NWSA Journal* 14, no. 2 (2002): 102-20. Accessed July 30, 2020.

Febles, Anthony John. "Rosenbergs Remembered in Sympathetic Exhibit." *Daily Collegian*, March 24, 1989.

Glueck, Grace. "Alice Neel, Self-Styled 'Collector of Souls,' Unfurls Her Own, in Glee and Heartbreak." *New York Times*, March 21, 1997, National edition, sec. C.

Harrison, Helen. "Art: Catching Corners of the Human Spirit." *New York Times*, May 4, 1986, National edition, sec. 11LI.

Hoban, Phoebe. *Alice Neel: The Art of Not Sitting Pretty*. New York: St. Martin's, 2010.

Kennaugh, Stuart. "Biography" Alice Neel, aliceneel.com.

Kino, Carol. "A Grandson Paints a Portrait of a Portraitist." *New York Times*, April 22, 2007.

Maine, Stephen. "Thriving on Drama and Discordance: The Life of Alice Neel." *artcritical*, August 3, 2011.

Neel, Alice, and Patricia Hills. *Alice Neel*. New York: H. N. Abrams, 1983.

Quinn, Bridget, and Lisa Congdon. *Broad Strokes: 15 Women Who Made Art and Made History (in That Order)*. San Francisco: Chronicle Books, 2017.

Schjeldahl, Peter. "Wild Life: Alice Neel's People." *New Yorker*, May 25, 2009.

Tasca, Cecilia, Mariangela Rapetti, Mauro Giovanni Carta, and Bianca Fadda. "Women and Hysteria in the History of Mental Health." *Clinical Practice & Epidemiology in Mental Health* 8, no. 1 (2012): 110-19.

ARTISTS AND SUICIDE

Andreasen, Nancy C. "The Relationship Between Creativity and Mood Disorders." *Dialogues in Clinical Neuroscience* 10, no. 2 (2008): 251-55. https://doi.org/10.31887/dcns.2008.10.2/ncandreasen.

Morrison, Ewan. "The Suicidal Artist." *Psychology Today*. Sussex Publishers, April 2, 2019. https://www.psychologytoday.com/us/blog/word-less/201904/the-suicidal-artist.

Sonke, Jill, Kelley Sams, Jane Morgan-Daniel, Andres Pumariega, Faryal Mallick, Virginia Pesata, and Nicola Olsen. "Systematic Review of Arts-Based Interventions to Address Suicide Prevention and Survivorship in Australia, Canada, the United Kingdom, and the United States of America." *Health Promotion Practice* 22, no. 1_suppl (2021). https://doi.org/10.1177/1524839921996350.

MARK ROTHKO

"Artist Mark Rothko." *American Masters Podcast*. Episode 37. PBS, October 29, 2019.

Baal-Teshuva, Jacob, and Mark Rothko. *Rothko*. Cologne: TASCHEN, 2015.

Breslin, James E. B. *Mark Rothko: A Biography*. Chicago: University of Chicago Press, 1998.

Chave, Anna, and Mark Rothko. *Mark Rothko: Subjects in Abstraction*. New Haven, CT: Yale University Press, 1989.

Cohen-Solal, Annie. *Mark Rothko: Toward the Light in the Chapel*. New Haven, CT: Yale University Press, 2015.

Cooke, Rachel. "The Art Cheats Who Betrayed My Father." *Guardian*, September 13, 2008. https://www.theguardian.com/artanddesign/2008/sep/14/art1.

Glueck, Grace. "Mark Rothko, Artist, a Suicide Here at 66." *New York Times*, February 26, 1970.

Güner, Fisun. "How Rothko Become the Mythic Superman of Mystical." *Abstraction* 1 (November 2014).

Hartman, JJ. "Risk Factors in Suicide: Mark Rothko and His Art." *Journal of Psychiatry and Mental Health* 3, no. 2 (2018). https://doi.org/10.16966/2474-7769.127.

Havelková, Tereza. "The Role of Myth in Mark Rothko's and Barnett Newman's Art." Bachelor's thesis, Charles University, 2016.

Jewell, Edward Alden. "'Globalism' Pops into View." *New York Times*, June 13, 1943.

Rothko, Mark, and Christopher Rothko. "Introduction." In *The Artist's Reality*, xi-xxxii. New Haven, CT: Yale University Press, 2004.

Seldes, Lee. *The Legacy of Mark Rothko*. New York: Da Capo, 1996.

Sheets, Hilarie M. "Mark Rothko's Dark Palette Illuminated." *New York Times*, November 3, 2016, sec. C.

JACOB LAWRENCE

Dickinson, Stephanie. *Jacob Lawrence: Painter*. New York: Cavendish Square, 2017.

Duggleby, John. *Story Painter: The Life of Jacob Lawrence*. San Francisco: Chronicle Books, 1998.

Figge Art Museum. "African American Art since 1950: Perspectives from the David C. Driskell Center." Teacher Resource Guide.

Hampton, Morgan. "Sedation [Jacob Lawrence]." Sartle.com.

Hills, Patricia, and Jacob Lawrence. *Painting Harlem Modern: The Art of Jacob Lawrence*. Berkeley: University of California Press, 2019.

National Gallery of Victoria. "Keith Haring | Jean-Michel Basquiat: Crossing Lines." Transcript of Multimedia Guide, narrated by Patti Astor. Victoria, Australia: National Gallery of Victoria, 2019.

Partridge, Erin. *Art Therapy with Older Adults: Connected and Empowered*. London: Jessica Kingsley, 2019.

Perry, Regenia A. "Free within Ourselves: African American Artists in the Collection of the National Museum of American Art." Smithsonian American Art Museum.

DIANE ARBUS

Bannon, Anthony. "The Biography Diane Arbus Always Deserved." *Buffalo News*, June 26, 2016.

Bosworth, Patricia. *Diane Arbus: A Biography*. New York: W. W. Norton, 2005.

Freud, Sigmund. *Beyond the Pleasure Principle*. London: International Psycho-Analytical Press, 1922.

Gerber, Alison Reppert. "Highlighting Diane Arbus: 'A Box of Ten Photographs.'" Smithsonian Institution Archives, March 29, 2018.

Lane, Anthony. "In the Picture: A New Biography of Diane Arbus." *New Yorker*, June 2016.

Leach, Diane. "Diane Arbus: 'Happiness Perplexed Her.'" *PopMatters*, February 21, 2020.

Lubow, Arthur, and Diane Arbus. *Diane Arbus: Portrait of a Photographer*. New York: Ecco, 2017.

Lubow, Arthur. "The Woman Who Influenced Diane Arbus's Eye." *Wall Street Journal*, May 25, 2016.

Mar, Alex. "The Cost of Diane Arbus's Life on the Edge." *The Cut*, July 12, 2016.

"Masters of Photography: Diane Arbus." Kent, Australia: Creative Arts Television Archive, Contemporary Arts Media (distributor), 1972.

Murtha, Tara. "'Diane Arbus': Genius? Predator? Is There a Difference?" *Philadelphia Inquirer*, September 4, 2016.

Nelson, Deborah. *Tough Enough: Arbus, Arendt, Didion, McCarthy, Sontag, Weil*. Chicago: University of Chicago Press, 2017.

O'Hagan, Sean. "Diane Arbus: Portrait of a Photographer Review—a Disturbing Study." *Guardian*, October 25, 2016.

Palumbo, Jacqui. "Revisiting Diane Arbus's Final and Most Controversial Series." *Artsy*, November 8, 2018.

Rexler, Lyle. "Through Her Lens Darkly: Diane Arbus's Life Was as Raw as Her Work." *New York Times*, July 1, 2016.

Ross, Jenna. "Diane Arbus: Purveyor Photographer of the Weird and Wacky." *TheCollector*, April 28, 2020.

Schultz, William Todd. *An Emergency in Slow Motion: The Inner Life of Diane Arbus*. New York: Bloomsbury, 2013.

Sehgal, Parul. "Diane Arbus's Sexual Adventures." *BookForum*, 2017.

Wender, Jessie. "The Subject of an Arbus." *New Yorker*, April 8, 2014.

Woodward, Richard B. "Diane Arbus: In the Park @Lévy Gorvy." *Collector Daily*, June 8, 2017.

WHAT IS TRAUMA?

Hoff, Ann. "'I Was Convulsed, Pitiably Hideous': Convulsive Shock Treatment in Leonora Carrington's Down Below." *Journal of Modern Literature* 32, no. 3 (2009): 83-98.

Salkaln, Elaine Mayers. "The Mystery Woman." *New York Times Magazine*, October 3, 2002.

GUSTAVE DORÉ

Church, F. P and W. C. Church. "Gustave Dore," *The Galaxy* 17 (1874): 344-53.

Cregan, Mary. *The Scar: A Personal History of Depression and Recovery*. New York: W. W. Norton, 2020.

Czapp, Patricia, and Kevin Kovach. "Poverty and Health—the Family Medicine Perspective (Position Paper)." American Academy of Family Physicians, 2015.

Evemy, Benjamin Blake. "Van Gogh's Asylum Year: The Sadness Will Last Forever." MutualArt, 2020.

Herendeen, W. H. "The Doré Controversy: Doré, Ruskin, and Victorian Taste." *Victorian Studies* 25, no. 3 (1982): 304-27.

Jerrold, Blanchard. "Introduction." In *London: A Pilgrimage*. Norwalk, CT: Easton, 2011.

Nochlin, Linda. *Misère: The Visual Representation of Misery in the 19th Century*. London: Thames and Hudson, 2018.

Norton, Frank H. *Paul Gustave Doré*. New York: J. B. Alden, 1883.

Popova, Maria. "Gustave Doré's Hauntingly Beautiful 1883 Illustrations for Edgar Allan Poe's 'The Raven.'" *Brain Picking*, January 19, 2016.

Roosevelt, Blanche. *Life and Reminiscences of Gustave Doré*. London: Sampson, 1885.

Saiber, Arielle, and Elizabeth Coggeshall. "Giuseppe De Liguoro, L'Inferno, 1911." Dante Today, July 11, 2017.

Wanamaker, Melissa. "Becoming Alexandra Styron." American Mental Health Foundation, May 1, 2015.

FRIDA KAHLO

Antelo, Fernando. "Pain and the Paintbrush: The Life and Art of Frida Kahlo." *American Medical Association Journal of Ethics* 15, no. 5 (May 2013): 460-65.

Bradley, Laura. "Frida Kahlo's Monkeys, Dogs & Birds." *AnOther*, October 13, 2011.

Bullen, Daniel. *The Love Lives of the Artists: Five Stories of Creative Intimacy*. Berkeley, CA: Counterpoint, 2011.

Chernick, Karen. "Frida Kahlo and Georgia O'Keeffe's Formative Friendship." *Artsy*, March 20, 2020.

Courtney, Carol A., Michael A. O'Hearn, and Carla C. Franck. "Frida Kahlo: Portrait of Chronic Pain." *Physical Therapy* 97, no. 1 (January 2017): 90-96.

Espinoza, Javier. "Frida Kahlo's Last Secret Finally Revealed." *Guardian*, August 11, 2007.

Fraley, R. Chris. "A Brief Overview of Adult Attachment Theory and Research." Department of Psychology University of Illinois at Urbana-Champaign, 2018.

Grimberg, Salomon. *Frida Kahlo: Song of Herself*. London: Merrell, 2008.

Herrera, Hayden. "Foreword." In *Frida Kahlo: Song of Herself*. By Salomon Grimberg, 11-32. London: Merrell, 2008.

Kahlo, Frida. "I'm Amputating You." *Letters of Note*, July 6, 2020.

Kettler, Sara. "Behind Frida Kahlo's Real and Rumored Affairs with Men and Women." Biography.com. A&E Networks Television, July 14, 2020.

Medina, Mariana, and Sara McIntosh Wooten. *Frida Kahlo: Self-Portrait Artist*. New York: Enslow, 2016.

Ochoa, Gerardo. "Biography of Frida Kahlo." Museo Frida Kahlo, June 2020.

Rocha, Lupe. "Kahlo's Reflection: The Absence of Equal Ability." *Medium*, July 27, 2018.

Souter, Gerry. *Frida Kahlo: Beneath the Mirror*. New York: Parkstone, 2005.

Stahr, Celia. *Frida in America: The Creative Awakening of a Great Artist*. New York: St. Martin's, 2020.

LEONORA CARRINGTON

Almino, Elisa Wouk. "The Idiosyncratic Writings of Leonora Carrington, a Reluctant Surrealist." *Hyperallergic*, June 20, 2017.

Butterworth, Lauren. "Leonora Carrington." *Deviant Women*, March 15, 2017.

Carrington, Leonora. *Down Below*. New York: New York Review of Books, 2017.

Carrington, Leonora. "Monday, 23 August 1943." In *Down Below*. New York: New York Review of Books, 2017.

Carrington, Leonora. "The Debutante." In *The Complete Stories of Leonora Carrington*. St. Louis, MO: Dorothy Project, 2017.

Chambers, Selena. "Hyenas, Horses, and Rabbits, Oh My! A Read Along Journey through the Leonora Carrington Century." *Weird Fiction Review*, June 16, 2017.

Crawford, Anwen. "Leonora Carrington Rewrote the Surrealist Narrative for Women." *New Yorker*, 2017.

Goodman, Justin. "*Down Below*, a Memoir by Leonora Carrington, Reviewed." *Cleaver Magazine*, June 18, 2020.

Hewison, James, and Michelle Man. *Leonora Carrington: Living Legacies*. Wilmington, DE: Vernon, 2020.

Hoff, Ann. "'I Was Convulsed, Pitiably Hideous': Convulsive Shock Treatment in Leonora Carrington's Down Below." *Journal of Modern Literature* 32, no. 3 (2009): 83-98.

Laity, Paul. "*The Surreal Life of Leonora Carrington* by Joanna Moorhead—Review." *Guardian*, April 5, 2017.

Leddy, Siobhan. "Why Surrealist Leonora Carrington Envisioned Women as Wild Animals." *Artsy*, May 4, 2019.

Moorhead, Joanna. "The Surrealist Muses Who Roared." *Guardian*, June 18, 2010.

National Museum of Women in the Arts. *Women in the Arts*, Summer 2006.

Rigg, Susannah. "Leonora Carrington Museum Is a Surreal Location for Surrealist Art." Gallery Wendi Norris, San Francisco, July 10, 2018.

Salkaln, Elaine Mayers. "The Mystery Woman." *New York Times*, October 13, 2002.

Schlatter, N. Elizabeth. "From the Collection: Leonora Carrington's Samhain Skin."

Sehgal, Parul. "The Romance and Heartbreak of Writing in a Language Not Your Own." *New York Times*, June 2, 2017.

Smith, Roberta. "Female Surrealists Re-emerge in 2 Startling Shows." *New York Times*, June 13, 2019.

Thackara, Tess. "The Market for Female Surrealists Has Finally Reached a Tipping Point." Gallery Wendi Norris, San Francisco, September 27, 2018.

Walsh, Joanna. "'I Have No Delusions. I Am Playing'—Leonora Carrington's Madness and Art." Versobooks.com, 2015.

Warner, Marina. "Introduction." In *Down Below*. By Leonora Carrington, vii-xxxiv. New York: New York Review of Books, 2017.

BODY IMAGE AND ART

Ganesan, Subhashini, SL Ravishankar, and Sudha Ramalingam. "Are Body Image Issues Affecting Our Adolescents? A Cross-Sectional Study among College Going Adolescent Girls." *Indian Journal of Community Medicine* 43, no. 5 (2018): 42. https://doi.org/10.4103/ijcm.ijcm_62_18.

Sotheby's. "Jenny Saville and the Beauty of Individualism." Sothebys.com. Sotheby's, February 18, 2019. https://www.sothebys.com/en/articles/jenny-saville-and-the-beauty-of-individualism.

YAYOI KUSAMA

Abrams, Loney. "Pop Art Ripoffs: The 3 Yayoi Kusama Artworks That Warhol, Oldenburg, and Samaras Copied in the '60s." *ArtSpace*, September 15, 2018.

Applin, Jo. *Yayoi Kusama: Infinity Mirror Room—Phalli's Field*. London: Afterall Books, 2012.

Karia, Bhupendra. *Yayoi Kusama: A Retrospective*. New York: Center for International Contemporary Arts, 1989.

Hoban, Phoebe. *Alice Neel: The Art of Not Sitting Pretty*. New York: St. Martin's, 2010.

Holmes, Helen. "Yayoi Kusama Just Published a Poem about the 'Terrible Monster' Coronavirus." *Observer*, April 15, 2020.

Hoptman, Laura J., Yayoi Kusama, Akira Tatehata, and Udo Kultermann. *Yayoi Kusama*. London: Phaidon, 2000.

Kusama: Infinity. Hulu, 2018.

Kusama, Yayoi, and Ralph F. McCarthy. *Infinity Net: The Autobiography of Yayoi Kusama*. London: Tate, 2020.

McCurry, Justin. "Justin McCurry Talks to Artist Yayoi Kusama." *Guardian*, June 5, 2009.

"Record-Breaking Kusama Leads Historical Contemporary Art Season in Asia." Sotheby's, May 9, 2019.

Romaine, James. "Yayoi Kusama's Infinity Nets: Sublime or Spectacle?" *Comment Magazine*, June 5, 2009.

Self-Obliteration. Shady Film Productions, 1967.

Taylor, Rachel. "Kusama's Relationship with Joseph Cornell." Tate.org, 2012.

INSTITUTIONAL RACISM AND TRAUMA

"The Body Remembers." Heather Agyepong, Multidisciplinary Artist//Actor, 2021. http://www.heatheragyepong.com/the-body-remembers.

Johanson, Christabel. "Mental Health in Black Art." africanah.org, September 7, 2020. https://africanah.org/mental-health-in-black-art/.

Weber, Jasmine. "A Portrait of Black Mental Health in Hues of Black and Blue."Hyperallergic, July 12, 2019. https://hyperallergic.com/469609/a-portrait-of-black-mental-health-in-hues-of-black-and-blue/.

JEAN-MICHEL BASQUIAT

"10 Things You Should Know about Dual Diagnosis Treatment." Dual Diagnosis.org, 2012.

"Are You Self-Medicating & Masking Symptoms of Mental Illness?" American Addiction Centers, 2020.

Brown, Nathan. "The Irony of Anatomy: Basquiat's Poetics of Black Positionality." *Radical Philosophy* 195 (2016).

Davis, Tamra, dir. *Jean-Michel Basquiat: The Radiant Child*. DVD. New York: Arthouse Films, 2011.

DeAngelis, Tori. "The Legacy of Trauma." *Monitor on Psychology* 50, no. 2 (February 2019): 36.

"Dual Diagnosis." National Alliance on Mental Illness, March 2015.

"East Village Art—Important Paintings." The Art Story. Accessed December 22, 2020.

Fanelli, James. "Jean-Michel Basquiat's Dad Leaves Behind Son's Art, and Tax Problem." DNAinfo. New York, September 5, 2013.

Faughnan, Ally. "The Best, Worst, and Weirdest Parts of Warhol and Basquiat's Friendship." *Dazed Digital*, May 28, 2019.

Foston, Nikitta. "Behind the Pain Nobody Talks About: Sexual Abuse of Black Boy." *Ebony* 58, no. 8 (June 2003).

Haden-Guest, Anthony. "Burning Out." *Vanity Fair*, November 1988.

Hays, Constance L. "Friends Recall Young Artist with Music and Verse." *New York Times*, November 6, 1988, sec. 1.

Hays, Constance L. "Jean Basquiat, 27, an Artist of Words and Angular Images." *New York Times*, August 15, 1988, sec. D.

Hoban, Phoebe. *Basquiat: A Quick Killing in Art*. New York: Viking, 1998.

hooks, bell. "Altars of Sacrifice: Re-membering Basquiat." In *Race-ing Art History: Critical Readings in Race and Art History*. Edited by Kymberly N. Pinder, 341-50. New York: Routledge, 2002.

Jagernauth, Kevin. "Jim Jarmusch Explains Why He Refuses to Watch Julian Schanbel's 'Basquiat.'" *IndieWire*, May 7, 2014.

Marshall, Richard. *Jean-Michel Basquiat*. New York: Whitney Museum of American Art, 1992.

McGuigan, Cathleen. "New Art, New Money." *New York Times Magazine*, March 17, 1985, sec. 6.

Raynor, Vivien. "Art: Basquiat, Warhol." *New York Times*, September 20, 1985, sec. C.

Raynor, Vivien. "Art: Paintings by Jean Michel Basquiat at Boone." *New York Times*, May 11, 1984, sec. C.

Rich, Motoko, and Robin Pogrebin. "Why Spend $110 Million on a Basquiat? 'I Decided to Go for It,' Japanese Billionaire Explains." *New York Times*, May 26, 2017, sec. C, p. 1.

"Phillips De Pury & Company Is Proud to Present to the Market Jean-Michel Basquiat's Seminal Painting from 1981 'Irony Of Negro Policeman.'" Phillips Auctioneers press release, June 8, 2012.

Schjeldahl, Peter. "Basquiat's Memorial to a Young Artist Killed by Police." *New Yorker*, July 2019.

Sloan, Aisha Sabatini. "On Basquiat, the Black Body, and a Strange Sensation in My Neck." *Paris Review*, October 26, 2017.

Traynor, Cian. "How Al Diaz and Jean-Michel Basquiat Rewrote the Rules of Street Art." *Huck Magazine*, February 12, 2019.

Wines, Michael. "Jean Michel Basquiat: Hazards of Sudden Success and Fame." *New York Times*, August 27, 1988, sec. 1.

Xhoxhi, Martin. "'Irony of Negro Policeman' by Basquiat, in Postmodernist Terms." *FAEM Martin Xhoxhi*, October 14, 2020.

GENDER IDENTITY AND DYSPHORIA

Dhejne, Cecilia, Roy Van Vlerken, Gunter Heylens, and Jon Arcelus. "Mental Health and Gender Dysphoria: A Review of the Literature." *International Review of Psychiatry* 28, no. 1 (2016): 44-57. https://doi.org/10.3109/09540261.2015.1115753.

Treaster, Joseph B. "Overlooked No More: Claude Cahun, Whose Photographs Explored Gender and Sexuality." *New York Times*, June 19, 2019. https://www.nytimes.com/2019/06/19/obituaries/claude-cahun-overlooked.html

WHAT IS "OUTSIDER ART"?

Rainaldi, Linda. 2015. "Outsider Art : Forty Years Out." Electronic Theses and Dissertations (ETDs) 2008+. T, University of British Columbia.

Schuster, Clayton. "In NYC, a Fair Dedicated to Outsider Art Cultivates an Interest in the Eccentric." *Observer*, 2020.

Steiner, Wendy. "In Love with the Myth of the 'Outsider.'" *New York Times*, March 10, 1996.

RICHARD DADD

Arnheim, Rudolf. "The Art of Psychotics." *Art Psychotherapy* 4, nos. 3-4 (1977): 113-20.

Banerjee, Jacqueline. "Sir Alexander Morison by Richard Dadd, 1817-1886." Victorian Web, June 27, 2020.

Bell, David. "Richard Dadd." Living with Schizophrenia, September 30, 2019.

Beveridge, Allan. "Richard Dadd: The Artist and the Asylum, by Nicholas Tromans." *British Journal of Psychiatry* 200, no. 4 (2012): 349-50.

Byatt, AS. "Richard Dadd: The Fairy King." *Guardian*, September 2, 2011.

Conliffe, Ciaran. "Richard Dadd, Artist and Mentally Disturbed Killer." HeadStuff, August 17, 2018.

Davidson, Jonathan. "Richard Dadd and *The Fairy Feller's Master-Stroke*." *American Journal of Psychiatry* 172, no. 11 (2015): 1073-74.

Doyle, Derek. "Sir Alexander Morison (1779-1866)." *Journal of the Royal College of Physicians of Edinburgh* 41, no. 4 (2011): 378.

Fowle, Frances. "'The Fairy Feller's Master-Stroke,' Richard Dadd, 1855-64." Tate, 2000.

Gaiman, Neil. "The Fairy Feller's Master Stroke." *Neil Gaiman's Journal*, January 1, 1970.

A Handbook to the Water Colours, Drawings, and Engravings in the Art Treasures Exhibition: Being a Reprint of Critical Notices Originally Published in "The Manchester Guardian." London: Bradbury and Evans, 1857.

Huddleston, Samuel, and G. A. Russell. "Richard Dadd: The Patient, the Artist, and the 'Face of Madness.'" *Journal of the History of the Neurosciences* 24, no. 3 (2015): 213-28.

Irving, Carolina, Miguel Flores-Vianna, and Charlotte Di Carcaci. "Bohemian Rhapsody." *New York Times*, February 10, 2015.

Morison, Alexander. *The Blackhalls of That Ilk and Barra, Hereditary Coronies and Foresters of the Garioch*. Aberdeen, Scotland: New Spalding Club, 1905.

Pearce, J. M. S. " Richard Dadd: Art and Madness." *Hektoen International* 11, no. 4 (2019).

Prodger, Michael. "The Dangerous Mind of Richard Dadd." *New Statesman*, July 2, 2015.

Sarnoff, Charles A. *Symbols in Structure and Function*. Vol. 3, *Symbols in Culture, Art, and Myth*. Bloomington, IN: Xlibris, 2003.

Scull, Andrew, Charlotte MacKenzie, and Nicholas Hervey. *Masters of Bedlam: The Transformation of the Mad-Doctoring Trade*. Princeton, NJ: Princeton University Press, 2014.

Seabrook, David. *All the Devils Are Here*. London: Granta, 2018.

"'The Flight out of Egypt,' Richard Dadd, 1849-50." Tate. Accessed January 4, 2021.

"Top 20 Finds on the *Antiques Roadshow*—Media Centre." BBC News. Accessed January 4, 2021.

Trainor, Terry. *Bedlam: St. Mary of Bethlehem*. Self-published, Lulu.com, 2010.

Tromans, Nicholas. "Richard Dadd: The Artist and the Asylum—TateShots." Tate, February 9, 2012.

Wood, William. *Remarks on the Plea of Insanity, and on the Management of Criminal Lunatics*. London: Longman, Brown, Green, and Longmans, 1851.

LOUIS WAIN

"Bethlem Museum of the Mind." Maudsley Charity, October 2, 2019.

Cardoso, Silvia Helena. "Cats Painted in the Progression of Psychosis of a Schizophrenic Artist." Neuroscience Art Gallery. Accessed September 21, 2020.

Coon, Dennis, and John O. Mitterer. *Introduction to Psychology: Gateways to Mind and Behavior*. Belmont, CA: Wadsworth: Cengage Learning, 2010.

The Curious Cats of Louis Wain. YouTube, 2018.

Denham, Sidney. "The Man Who Drew Cats: From the Archive, 5 August 1960." *Guardian*, August 5, 2013.

Gallagher, Paul. "The Psychedelic Madness of Louis Wain's Cats." DangerousMinds, May 29, 2016.

Haining, Peter, ed. *A Cat Compendium: The Worlds of Louis Wain*. London: Peter Owen, 2014.

Kennedy, Philip. "Cute Cats and Psychedelia: The Tragic Life of Louis Wain." *Illustration Chronicles*, November 2016.

Milton, Joseph. "How a Mental Disorder Opened Up an Invisible World of Colour and Pattern." *Scientific American*, December 22, 2011.

Moody, Paul. “The Forgotten Artist Who Changed the Way We Look at Cats.” *Another Man*, October 18, 2018.

Novara, Caterina, Gioia Bottesi, Stella Dorz, and Ezio Sanavio. “Hoarding Symptoms Are Not Exclusive to Hoarders.” *Frontiers in Psychology* 7 (November 2016).

O’Flynn, David. “Kaleidoscope Cats: A Clinical Perspective on Louis Wain.” YouTube. Lecture presented at the Bethlem Museum of the Mind, 2012.

Philo, Chris. “The Wild and Tranquil Geographies of Animals and Madness.” Edinburgh History of Medicine Group. Lecture presented at the Royal College of Physicians of Edinburgh, November 20, 2019.

Riggs, Ransom. “Did Cats Drive This Painter Insane?” *Mental Floss*, November 9, 2010.

Sorene, Paul. “Louis Wain: The Man Who Drew Millions of Far-Out Cats.” *Flashbak*, July 3, 2018.

Watson, Danielle, “Psychotic Diagnosis and Artist Pathology: Schizophrenic Art’s Influence on the Identification of the Disorder.” (2014). *Honors Projects*. 160.

Wehring, Heidi J., and William T. Carpenter. “Violence and Schizophrenia.” *Schizophrenia Bulletin* 37, no. 5 (September 2011): 877-78.

ALOÏSE CORBAZ

“Aloïse Corbaz, 1886-1964.” *Raw Vision*. Accessed November 18, 2020.

“The Art Brut of Aloïse Corbaz.” Schiz Life, January 12, 2016.

Delistraty, Cody. “The Art of Madness.” *Paris Review*, February 6, 2018.

Laird, Michele. “The Creative Schizophrenia of Aloïse.” SWI, November 6, 2017.

Muzelle, Céline. “The Art of Aloïse: A Lone Continent?” *Raw Vision*, Fall 2012.

Porret-Forel, Jacqueline. “Aloïse & the Theater of the Universe.” https://www.ubu.com

Prinzhorn, Hans. *Artistry of the Mentally Ill: A Contribution to the Psychology and Psychopathology of Configuration*. Eastford, CT: Martino Fine Books, 2019.

Ruoss, B. S. *The Subject of Schizophrenia—All You Want to Know about the Illness*. Bloomington, IN: Xlibris US, 2020.

Russell, Charles. “Aloïse Corbaz.” Outsider Art Fair. Accessed November 18, 2020.

Steiner, Wendy. “In Love with the Myth of the ‘Outsider.’” *New York Times*, March 10, 1996.

AGNES MARTIN

"Agnes Martin." Pace Gallery. Accessed November 18, 2020.

Als, Hilton. "The Heroic Art of Agnes Martin." *New York Review of Books*, July 14, 2016.

Cotter, Holland. "The Joy of Reading between Agnes Martin's Lines." *New York Times*, October 6, 2016, sec. C.

Gruen, John. "Agnes Martin: 'Everything, Everything Is about Feeling . . . Feeling and Recognition.'" *ARTnews*, 1976.

Harris, Jennifer. "Agnes Martin: MoMA." Museum of Modern Art, 2016.

Laing, Olivia. "Agnes Martin: The Artist Mystic Who Disappeared into the Desert." *Guardian*, May 22, 2015.

Martin, Agnes. *Writings*. Edited by Dieter Schwarz. Ostfildern, Germany: Edition Cantz, 1993.

Martin, Henry. *Agnes Martin: Pioneer, Painter, Icon*. Tucson, AZ: Schaffner, 2018.

Miranda, Carolina A. "Q&A: What the World Misunderstands about Artist Agnes Martin and How Her Biographer Unearthed Her Story." *Los Angeles Times*, April 12, 2016.

Princenthal, Nancy. *Agnes Martin: Her Life and Art*. London: Thames and Hudson, 2015.

"Seen in Context: Agnes Martin's Gabriel." Lévy Gorvy, April 5, 2019.

Weber, Joanna. "The House That Agnes Martin Built." *Image* 63 (2015).

Sartle.com is a project devoted to democratizing art history by focusing on the stories that textbooks often ignore. This book was made possible by Sartle, which mixes serious art history with snarky observations and hilarious, strange, and shocking facts about artworks and artists, making art more relatable and fun.
>> www.sartle.com

Kathryn Vercillo is a full-time writer with a master's degree in psychological studies. She is the owner of Create Me Free, a small business that researches the link between art and mental health in order to educate, inspire, and empower artists to achieve financial and creative success while maintaining wellbeing. She is the author of eight books, including *Crochet Saved My Life*, which is about the health benefits of handcrafting. When not creating, she's enjoying life in San Francisco with her loved ones and her rescue pups.

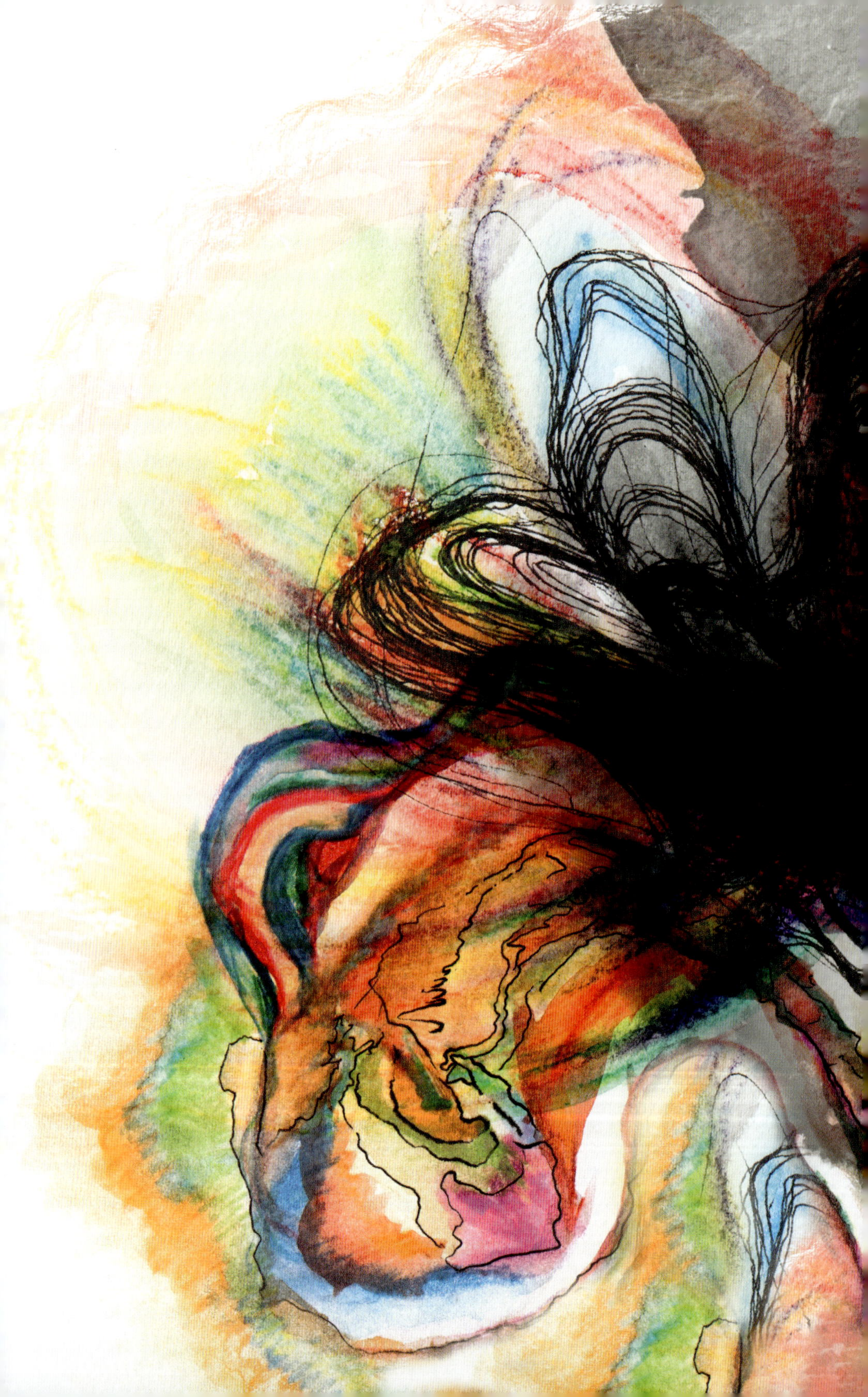

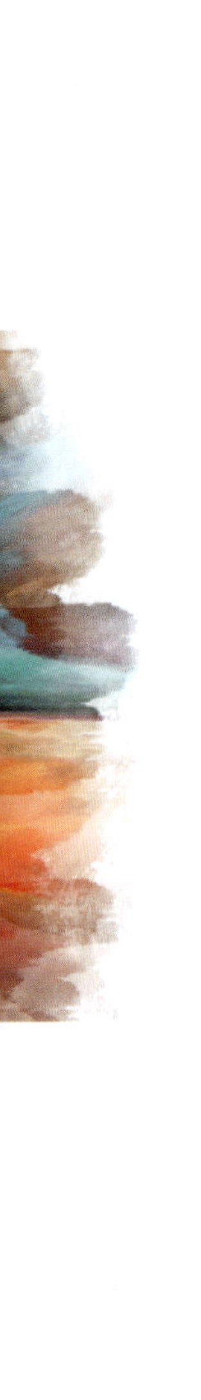